# Make Your Own Essential Oils from Raw Plants

## Using Oils & Herbs for Optimum Health

By **Amber Richards**

# Table of Contents

Introduction .................................................................................. 1

Essences ...................................................................................... 3

Essential Oils .............................................................................. 5

The History of Essential Oils ..................................................... 9

Essential Oils as Antiseptics ..................................................... 13

Many Other Uses for Essential Oils ......................................... 19

Essential Oils and Means of Administration ........................... 27

Gathering and Preserving Aromatic Plants ............................. 29

Infusions or Decoctions ............................................................ 35

Plant Preparation: Definition, Methods And Its Uses ............ 37

Essential Oils and Some of Their Uses .................................... 43

Make Your Own Essential Oils ................................................ 69

Preparing Your Medicine Chest ............................................... 73

Which Part of the Herb is Used? .............................................. 77

Preparations of Essential Oil Capsules, Salves, Syrups and Tinctures .................................................................................... 91

Essential Oils For Beauty Treatments ................................... 105

Essential Oils For Tonics and Teas ........................................ 113

Conclusion ............................................................................... 123

# Introduction

Taking care of our health is an important goal in life. Anyone who has faced health challenges knows this should not ever be taken for granted. Learning strategies and methods that can help us reach optimum levels of health not only will benefit us now, but surely in years to come as well. We desire that our 'golden years' be ones in which we are strong and healthy enough to enjoy, until the end of our lives ideally.

In this book we'll be looking at various herbs and essential oils in the role of increasing our overall health and hopefully, overcome in a natural way health challenges we may be facing. There are many methods for using plants and their oils, and we'll also be showing how you can make your own essential oils (which can be expensive to purchase), from raw plants.

It is interesting to be familiarized with the various types of medicine that human beings have developed for their fellow men since the beginning. From time to time, we find ourselves brought back to the era of simple and ordinary natural medicine, if indeed we have ever completely abandoned it. Most often we return to it as a last resort, when some serious condition has failed to respond to the whole gamut of modern therapies. We should obviously do better and waste less time if, for a number of diseases, we made it our starting point.

Recent discoveries, such as those which have shown the existence of hormones and antibiotic principles in many plants and essences, suggest that we should have been wary of making snap judgments about how such medicines work. We have now been given a simple and logical account of their action, through various hormonal correspondences, on both the physical body and the psyche.

Numerous experiments enable us to explain some of the age-old treatments which, until now, were dismissed with a smile - a sachet of garlic or other plants, for instance, which our forefathers used to hang around the necks of children plagued with worms, or used more generally during epidemic outbreaks.

And yet the informed use of plants and essences can produce effects, which to the layman appear nearly miraculous. The Ancient Egyptians already knew how to anesthetize subjects with full-bodied maceration of plants.

The names of the most eminent researchers, doctors, biologists and pharmacists continually appear among the authors of the numerous works that deal with plants and essential oils.

Normal preventive medicine, which consists of giving healthy people drugs and injections of products whose future effects are unpredictable, can make some feel cautious. More and more people are turning to more natural methods.

# Essences

Essences are usually obtained by the distillation of the plants, and, in the case of most of the plants considered, are generally prescribed in the form of drops, pearls or capsules. Separate sections for garlic, onion and chamomile are intentionally separated for these are practically never prescribed by doctors. Why? It is because the action of these plants and seasonings are partly due to their aromatic essences.

Very often, an effective method of treatment involves no more than daily use in the kitchen of garlic, clove, sage, rosemary, thyme, savory and many other herbs or seasonings. Apart from infusions, powders, fumigations, liniments and baths achieve their effects by means of the volatile oils they release.

In spite of the rare problems encountered with the use of plants and essences, "Doctors and chemists will be surprised at the wide range of odoriferous substances which may be used medicinally," wrote R.M. Gattefosse (considered to be the Father of Aromatherapy), who added "And at the great variety of their chemical functions." Besides the antiseptic and anti-microbial properties of which use is currently made, the essential oils are also anti-toxic and anti-viral; they have a powerful energizing effect and possess an undeniable cicatrizing property.

To continue, when the object is to analyze an aromatic essence intended for consumption (they generally carry the label "pure and natural" on the authority of the manufacturer when they are often adulterated), the chromatographic method is used to examine the succession of peaks obtained on a moving graph. You would expect it to be sufficient to compare the "curve" with the image type given by the truly pure and natural essence as reference.

Go to one of these control laboratories one day, and you will observe that, alongside the machine which is supposed to be infallible, there is always a "nose" - i.e., a man or woman of highly specialized skills, who for every individual graph, will always sniff at the vapor which is given off. It is the "nose" which says "the apparatus is right", or if not, will correct the information given.

Generally speaking, plants, whether used fresh or in powder form, in infusions or decoctions, internally or externally by means of fumigations, liniments, poultices or baths, come up to expectation - so long at these important conditions are met: they must be picked at the right moment and in a predetermined place; they must be dried and preserved with skill to keep the power intact, and they must be used with discrimination.

The medicinal use of aromatic essences, otherwise known as plant essences, essential oils or volatile oils, has a long tradition. However, in spite of a great deal of scientific investigation, the method of action is still not precisely known, but this in no way diminishes their therapeutic value. In contrast to many modern medicines, with rare exceptions, and then only when used on patients with some particular predisposition (like an allergy), neither plants nor their essences cause repercussions or complications. This provides an excellent reason, if more is needed, for turning to them.

Through the ages, most centuries developed new plant formulas and recipes. For instance, the Romans grew aromatic herbs, Egypt developed embalming compounds with essences and resins, the Greeks were adept with perfumes and Babylon had special orange flower baths to be enjoyed.

# Essential Oils

Aromatic essences are oily and fragrant substances that can be found from plants in such a diversity of ways: by form of pressing (e.g. cloves), by form of tapping (laurel), by form of separation with the use of heat (turpentine), and there are some cases where solvents are used, or with effleurage (circular, stroking massage).

Essential oils are most often present in smaller quantities when compared with the plant mass. The normal method of the distillation procedure is very similar to that used in the production of distilled water; however, the same water must be distilled with further quantities of the substances, since if this is not done a considerable quantity of essence will be lost.

Certain types of these essential oils do appear in the pharmacopoeia of the world. In France, the 1949 edition - Codex VII - contains about fifteen. Earlier editions contained many more, twenty-four in 1937, forty-four in 1837.

Aromatic essences in general pre-existed in plants, though there are some which form only with the presence of water.

Though generally colorless, a few essences are distinctively colored, as detailed here: the essence of cinnamon, for instance, is reddish; the essence of chamomile, blue and the essence of wormwood, green. Some (e.g. the essences of bitter almonds, cinnamon and garlic) are heavier than water, but most are lighter, most essences are liquids, some are solids.

Essences are to be distinguished from fatty oils, which are fixed and will stain a paper permanently, in that they are volatized by heat and their stain is temporary. They are soluble in alcohol, ether and fixed oils yet insoluble in water, to which they nevertheless impart their scent.

Their boiling points vary from 160 degrees to 240 degrees Celsius and their densities from 0.759 to 1.096. They dissolve grease, iodine, sulfur and phosphorous. They reduce certain salts. They are stimulants which can be used both internally and externally, usually in a solution of alcohol or another suitable solvent. They are also perfumes.

There was a time when essences were considered to be definite substances. But with the birth of the science of organic chemistry at the end of the nineteenth century, they gradually began to yield up their secrets, even though today all has not yet been discovered about them. A professor from the University of Austin, Texas has observed that essences present more new compounds than the chemists of the whole world could analyze in a thousand years. At least we now know that they are mixtures of many constituents, such as the following: terpenes, alcohols, esters, aldehydes, ketones and phenols, to name a few.

According to their elementary composition:

1. Hydrocarbon essences, i.e. those rich in terpenes (e.g. the essences of turpentine and lemon); these are the most numerous.
2. Oxygenized essences (e.g. the essences of rosé and mint); these are generally solid essences.
3. Sulphureted essences (the Cruciferae and Liliaceae).

Many essences are a mixture of carbides and oxygenized substances in which one finds most of the chemical functions of organic matter. The following are some examples: hydrocarbons or terpenes such as thymes, alcohols such as geraniol and linalol, aldehydes like the essences of bitter almonds and citral, esters like the acetates of bornyl and linalyl, ketones like carvone and thujone, and phenols like eugenol, thymol and carvacol.

Some essences whose composition have been clearly defined, or at least appears to have been, are reproduced synthetically; but there are good grounds for believing that the results obtained with synthetic essences cannot be compared with the effects of natural essential oils.

The quality of essential oils depends on many factors. The process by which the substance is obtained, its state of maturity and preservation and its source are all important. There are "prize localities" for certain essences, such as the following: Ceylon for cinnamon, the West Indies for lemongrass, and Reunion for Thyme, for example.

Essentials oils are often adulterated with alcohol, fixed oils, and essential oils of lesser value and certain synthetic esters; such as soap from animal fats or gelatin.

Finally, to be able to preserve these essences one should keep them in well-sealed containers away from air and light (use colored glass). It is vital to avoid oxidation, polymerisation and resinification, which will occur (and ruin your oils) if these precautions are not taken.

# The History of Essential Oils

When one considers the history of aromatic essences, one may go back thousands of years to find distillation of plants as they were practiced in ancient Persia, Turkey and India. Romans had the awareness of the Greek's process, who had received such from Egypt in turn. The Egyptians seem to have known how to prepare an essence of cedar wood. The way it worked was the wood was heated in a clay vessel with its opening covered by a screen of woolen fibers; the essence would then be obtained by squeezing out the impregnated wool.

The Arabs discovered the distilling of plants in the Middle Ages. In the thirteenth century, the new pharmaceutical industry encouraged the development of distillation, and about this time the Master Glovers were granted the right to saturate their gloves with perfume and to sell scented oils. The essence of rosemary was one of the first to be isolated at this time. In the sixteenth century, the perfume industry in Provence was producing essences of lavender and aspic. It was a trade that flourished; especially at Montpellier, Narbonne and Grasse.

The aromatic essences of aspic, bitter almond, cedar, cinnamon, frankincense, juniper, mastic, rose and sage were all known by about the fifteenth century. During the next hundred years, sixty more essences came to be added to the list, and included aloes, angelica, aniseed, basil, bay, bryony, chamomile, cardamom, caraway, celery, cloves, coriander, cumin, fennel, galingale, ginger, guaiacum, hyssop, lavender, mace, melissa, myrrh, nutmeg, orange, origanum, parsley, pepper, peppermint, rue, saffron, sandalwood, savory, sassafras, sweet marjoram, tansy, thyme and wild thyme. By the beginning of the 17$^{th}$ Century, with the isolation of the essences of artemisia, bergamot, boxwood, cajuput, chervil, cypress, mustard, orange-flower, pine, savin, thuja and valerian among others, most of the useful essences of Europe and the near East had been discovered.

In France at the time of Louis XIV it was considered good form to take an interest in concoctions of essences which bore one's own name. There was a powder "a la Marechale" named after the Marechale d'Aumont. Any number of perfumes, creams and cosmetics were dressed up with the family name of one of the great lords or ladies. But the general lack of hygiene led to such an abuse of perfumes that towards the end of his reign the Sun King simply forbade them.

From the 18th Century onwards, attempts were made to control the adulteration of essential oils. This was the time when Feminis created the "eau admirable", later to be called "Eau de Cologne". A nephew, Farina, established a house in Paris to market the product.

With the 19th Century came the first analyses. From 1818 onwards, it was well known that all terpenic hydrocarbons were in the constant proportion of five carbon atoms to eight hydrogen atoms. In 1825, Boulet discovered cumarin. Kekule coined the name "terpene" in 1866, and the following year benzoic aldehyde was prepared for the first time by a chemical process. Perkin synthesized cumarin in 1868, and in 1876, in the rue Saint Charles in Paris, G. de Laire founded the first factory for the synthetic preparation of perfumes. 1822 saw the establishing of the constitution of eugenol, a fundamental element of the essence of cloves; the first artificial musk was produced in 1887. Clearly we are no longer in the infancy of things synthetic and artificial; the first steps into the chemical era have been taken. It is since that time that Western man has begun to use chemical colorings and preservatives in food.

A number of essences have established reputations; some have already acquired the patents of nobility - citral and linalol, for instance, whose composition had been studied since 1980.

Surely we should be filled with admiration, and humbled too, as we discover how accurate the information was about plants and essences that the ancients possessed and how effective their application of that knowledge was. When we consider that reaching the same point ourselves has required so much research and experimentation, often of a complex and delicate nature demanding highly sophisticated equipment. In this whole field we find, as a general principal, that we can add little to what has been handed down to us. We must recognize the fact that our forefathers were correct. Goethe (German statesman and writer in the 1800s) once wrote: "In my own canton there were wise men who could read no more than their breviary".

It is conceivable that the day will come when the true therapeutic value of natural substances will be given their proper recognition.

# Essential Oils as Antiseptics

Since it was discovered that they are rich in terpenes and phenols, alcohols and aldehydes, natural essences have been regarded as endowed with antiseptic properties, though in fact their bactericidal action has been established in practice for hundreds of years.

There is a relationship between the bactericidal power of essential oils and their chemical function. In order of decreasing potency we have phenols, aldehydes, alcohols, esters and acids (opinions still differing with regard to the terpenes). These constituents generally have greater antiseptic properties than synthetic phenol.

Since the chemical nature of the essences are varied, while their antiseptic power is general, it is thought that this property common to essences must be attributed to common physical traits. Some authors hold that the disinfectant action of essences is proportional to a reduction in the surface tension; others that it is attributable to special solubility on the limiting film of living cells.

The antiseptic action has been determined both in the presence of essence vapors and in direct contact with essential oils.

The first research into the antiseptic powers of essential oils was undertaken by Chamberland in 1887, in his work on the anthrax bacillus. He noted the active properties of origanum, Chinese cinnamon, Singhalese cinnamon, Angelica and Alferian geranium.

The antigenic potency of essences in their state of being vaporized appears in an increasing order: Chinese anise, eucalyptus, sandalwood, rosemary, peppermint, niaouli, lavender, citronella, clove, juniper, bergamot, orange, thyme, and lemon. Such order parallels almost exactly with the strong point of essence being studied in relation to the terpenes.

The antigenic properties of these vapors are experienced above in relation to meningococcus, staphylococcus and the typhus bacillus. The diphtheria bacillus is much more resistant, and the spores of the anthrax bacillus were not affected at all.

The decreasing order of anti-genetic activity in essential oils is slightly different in the case of direct contact: thyme, lemon, juniper, peppermint, niaouli, eucalyptus, sandalwood, anise, Chinese anise.

The essences of eucalyptus, clove, niaouli, thyme, garlic, sandalwood, lemon, cinnamon, lavender, German chamomile and peppermint are particularly notable for their antiseptic properties, and some of these deserve to be sifted out for closer attention.

The essence of eucalyptus is sometimes replaced by its chief constituent, eucalyptol. This substance is used in an oily solution (5 to 10g %) as a nasal application and is also given in intra-muscular injections. Internally, it is administered in 0.2g capsules. Some researchers, however, give the leading role to the terpenic carbides which eucalyptus contains, and to them eucalyptol appears to be a lifeless substance.

Clove essence kills tuberculosis bacillus at a certain strength ranging from one part up to six thousand. In dentistry it is used as a disinfectant and cauterizing agent, though for this purpose it is being increasingly replaced by its principal constituent, eugenol. An essence's antiseptic power is used with a dilution of one percent; it's still three to four times that more active compared to that of phenol.

The essence of niaouli is used in a 5 to 10 % oily solution, to soothe wounds, burns or ulcers. Niaouli water is also used, in a 2% percent solution. It is prepared by shaking, and is taken internally in the form of capsules of niaouli at 50% (1g per day). Niaouli has traditionally been used in New Caledonia, its inhabitants eating the leaves, making infusions and using the essence to disinfect water.

Thyme is an exceptional antiseptic on account of the thymol that it contains. Much has already been written on the peroxidized essence's bactericidal power. The watery solution at five percent kills typus bacillus (a typhoid fever) and also Shiga's bacillus (epidemic dysentery agent) in two minutes. It can also kill colon bacillus in just a short time of two to eight minutes, streptococcus as well as diphtheric bacillus in about four minutes, the staphylococcus in four to eight minutes, and the tuberculosis bacillus from thirty to sixty minutes. With the strength of about 0.1 %, thyme's peroxidized essence is in a form of diluted solution with soapy water that destroys the microbial flora of the mouth within three minutes.

The essence of garlic is used in a preventive capacity during influenza epidemics, and as a modifier of bronchial secretions.

Sandalwood's essence is very distinct for disinfecting the urinary tract, and is generally taken with 0.25g of capsules. Other kinds of essences are powerful too, in disinfecting the urinary tract, particular juniper, turpentine and lavender.

Lemon's essence is second to none, for its bactericidal and antiseptic properties. Morel and Rochaix's works have clearly demonstrated lemon essence's vapors can neutralize meningococcus in just fifteen minutes, typhus bacillus within not more than an hour, pneumococcus in one to three hours, staphylococcus aureus in two.

Alone, the essence can neutralize typhus bacillus in just five minutes and in twenty minutes the diphtheric bacillus also. A few drops of lemon can rid an oyster of about 92% of its micro-organisms in 15 minutes.

The astonishing antiseptic power of an aromatic essence is a well-established fact. We can find it used in everyday products such as toothpaste, where the efficacy of anise, clove, chamomile, peppermint and other essential oils as a base is undisputed. Even the addition of the best known bactericidal agents has done nothing to increase the antiseptic power of toothpaste made from these essences. It is quite understandable that, rather than using chemical products which may be dangerous or ineffective against germs, manufacturers will time and again choose natural essences.

In the past, when the composition of essential oils was a mystery, even without understanding the chemical processes involved, people were able to benefit from their antiseptic properties; whether in the form of food (garlic, onion, etc.), or vapors for the prevention and control of epidemics.

The antiseptic properties of aromatic essences are put to good use every day by the person who uses garlic, thyme, lemon, cloves and other spices, in the kitchen on a regular basis.

There are a variety of ways in which essential oils can be administered: internally, singly or in combination, and generally as pills, or drops in an alcoholic solution; externally chiefly as fumigations, inhalations, liniments and general or localized baths. Aromatic essential oils are among the most effective bath additives. Many studies have shown the transformation which may be caused in this way, both physically and psychologically, by their action upon the nervous system, the alimentary canal, the urinary tract, and their hormonal influence. These effects which result from the extraordinary diffusibility of the essences, suggest a logical explanation for the ancient practice of hanging a little bag of garlic cloves around the necks of children suffering with worms, or wearing such a bag as a protection against epidemic diseases.

Some soaps can emulsify essential oils, and the resulting preparations are extremely useful for bathing wounds. Where moist dressings are needed for the treatment of boils, abscesses, lymphangitis, burns, gangrenous or cancerous wounds and leg ulcers, their germ killing and healing action has been shown highly superior to that of oxygenated water, formalin, or Dakin's liquor, a common treatment today for suppurating wounds. The aromatic substances that become soluble in water by means of a suitable "softener" may be used in the same way.

Essential oils are also valuable as antiseptics because of their aggressiveness towards the microbial germs are being matched with the harmlessness to the body's tissue. One of the chief defects of chemical antiseptics is that they can be as harmful to the cells of the body, as the cause of the disease is.

The scent of essential oils does not cover up the bad smells of infected gangrenous or cancerous wounds; it suppresses them by physico-chemical action. The resins and essences used in the embalming of bodies prevent putrefaction. The Egyptians knew this; many butchers as well, for they use aromatics to prevent their meat from rotting.

There seems to be two major types of biological reactions: synthesis, whose processes give rise to forms generally characterized by sweet aromas, and degradation, whose processes are generally characterized by offensive, and in the case of rotten meat and eggs, for instance, repulsive smells. Illness is a process of degradation which precedes decomposition, and here aromatic essences have their benefit in that they can hinder this process while promoting the decomposition, digestion and neutralization of germs.

Surely this is a key factor: the antiseptic power of essences does not diminish nor become blunted with the passing of time. Why not? It is hard to find a satisfactory answer, but perhaps it is because these natural substances, besides jugulating infections, reinforce the body's own defense mechanisms. They are in fact powerful alternatives. Furthermore, the body does not appear to become accustomed to aromatherapy in the way that it does to synthetic sleeping pills, for instance, or in the case of body and germs, resistant to the forms of treatments using antibiotics.

# Many Other Uses for Essential Oils

Besides their antiseptic and bactericidal properties, many essential oils have antiviral properties as well.

Shingles, caused by a filterable virus, is generally painful and begins with violent attacks of neuralgia, often localized on the left or right side of the thorax, or equally on the left or right hemi-face (ophthalmic shingles, may lead to the loss of an eye), sometimes extending to the arm. It is characterized by an eruption of vesicles reminiscent of herpes arranged in groups along the path of the sensitive nerves of the skin, always on one side of the body only. Normally accompanied by severe pain, they evolve into ulcers. The localization of shingles on the nervous system has caused the condition to be called "posterior poliomyelitis". It can develop in a very serious way, the ulceration leading to extensive sores which are very painful and tenacious.

At the moment there is no specific treatment for shingles and it is still often treated with soothing ointments and, not very convincingly, the ingestion of vitamins and the use of X-rays. A mixture of essential oils can suppress shingles in about a week if the condition is treated during the first days of its occurrence (a little more time is required if the condition has already developed).

Influenza is also caused by a filterable virus, which by itself gives rise to a harmless cold, but in association with various microbes may lead to bronchi-pulmonary conditions with varying degrees of seriousness, depending on the patient and the outbreak. It is a fact that every year the "flu" is responsible for several thousand deaths.

Many essences (e.g. cinnamon, pine needles, thyme, lemon) have marked effects on these conditions, and patients treated with these essences for a variety of complaints seem to get through the winter without much trouble.

The antiseptic power of these essences is complemented by their cicatrizing properties. Found chiefly among the Labiatae (e.g. lavender, sage, thyme, rosemary), these properties can assist in the healing of abrasions or infected wounds, leg ulcers and fistulas. The essences have this healing effect because of their ability to increase the blood supply to the tissue, and this assists both the detergent action of the white corpuscles and cell regeneration. Aromatic wines, which were so prevalent at the time of the Renaissance, had an excellent reputation in this respect and numerous writings stressed their value in the treatment of burns, abrasions and infected wounds. Gangrenous wounds may also be treated successfully with essential oils. Acting as powerful disinfectants, they bring about a true embalming process which leads to cicatrization.

When aromatic essences are used, healing takes place quickly and without dangerous toxicity or the formation of scars. Some essential oils in fact, have quite startling effects on reducing old, keloid or unsightly scars.

A fragrant smell is as much a factor in health as it is in beauty, and part of the curative effect of essences may be seen in the subtle change in odor which they bring about, for this is normally an indication of structural change. The idea is confirmed in practice. Take, for instance, the example of phenols and alcohols. Phenols possess the property of attaching themselves to the amino-acids which cause the destructive action of numerous microbial germs or their secretions, as well as tissue waste in wounds, burns, and skin conditions. The resulting products (aminophenols) are well known for their antiseptic action, in fact, this is one of the explanations of the bactericidal actions of phenols. Alcohols behave in a similar fashion, producing amino-alcohols. Amino-menthol and other amino-alcohols have been linked with certain substances which are active in regard to the leprosy bacillus, parent of the tubercle bacillus, and this would explain the effect of menthol on bronchial patients.

We have already considered the healing power of aromatic essences in relation to burns and wounds, in that they encourage the reconstruction of damaged tissue. Skin diseases also will sometimes respond to treatment with essential oils. Lesions of this kind are always a sign of a poor organic condition and indicate abnormality in the composition of the layers of the skin and the presence of an element of decay. Besides halting the decay, the essences may encourage a synthesis, which leads to the reconstruction of the tissue. The various dermatoses (wet or dry), acne and blotches are curable by both local and general treatment with essential oils. Local application of essences also acts upon the subjacent organ (liver, intestine circulatory system) whose deficiency has given rise to the skin problem.

Apart from citral (either in ointment form or injected), and various pastes which may be neutral or acidic, there are certain combinations of flower essences (from both indigenous and exotic flowers) which may be used in the treatment of eczema and indeed a variety of skin conditions, particularly acne, certain types of psoriasis, "bricklayers' itch" and the butterfly mask of pregnancy. While such essences as mustard, cinnamon, clove, turpentine, pine and cypress are strongly rubefacient, the majority have only a slight irritant action on the skin and deterpenated essences none at all.

The pesticidal properties of essences have also been known about for ages. The essences of lavender, geranium and oregano, among others, will repel insects including moths and mosquitoes and are wonderfully effective in the treatment of insect bites, spider bites and wasp stings.

In fact, most essences have anti-toxic and anti-venomous properties as well. In the case of these bites and stings, if one has no bottle of essential oil on hand, an excellent substitute treatment is to rub the affected parts with the flowers of lavender, rosemary, sage leaves, a cut leek, a piece of onion, or garlic. The pain quickly disappears, and the inflammation fades away within a few minutes (one should not forget to remove a wasp's stinger of course). These essences neutralize the insect venom.

Many essential oils have anti-neuralgic and anti-rheumatic properties when applied to a localized area in the form of emulsions, ointments, liniments or compresses. This knowledge has been used for centuries; in the past people used applications of plants they heated in the oven for poultices of garlic, onion, thyme and sage to treat painful rheumatic conditions and gout.

The anti-rheumatic properties are released by external use and act on a particular area. But the large scale diffusion of essences through the skin suggests that the treatment also works internally. Juniper baths are recommended for people suffering from rheumatism or arthritis; baths of marjoram, thyme, rosemary or sage are fortifying, baths of lavender are soothing, as are baths of lime flowers.

The skin's absorptive nature has always been used in the treatment of general conditions (e.g. with iodine paint or rubbing with liniments based in garlic, olive oil or camphor). The modern pharmacopoeia contains many ointments whose active principle (anti-coagulant or hormonal), is designed to have an effect on the whole body through rubbing into the skin.

If essences have this effect when applied to a local area of the skin, one wonders how powerfully they must act when taken internally. In fact their properties are varying and almost infinite when taken in this way.

They are found to be antiseptics (with regard to lungs, intestine and urinary tract), anti-ferments, detoxifiers, remineralizers, stimulants and antispasmodics (not in fact incompatible, since essences are usually balancing agents), diuretics, anti-rheumatics, digestives, carminatives, febrifuges, cholagogues and vermifuges. The majority have hormonal properties which act on the cortex of the suprarenal (adrenal) glands, ovaries and thyroid. Some are aphrodisiacs, while others have been shown to be vaso-dilators or vaso-constrictors, and to act against diabetes.

As a result of a great deal of research, we are now able to explain the action of essences on the intestinal motor function, their relations with the various endocrine glands, the manner in which they are eliminated and their vascular, analgesic and cell-protecting properties.

Among the antiseptics we may mention lemon, thyme, lavender, turpentine, pine, eucalyptus, clove, etc.; in fact, the list is almost endless. In the treatment of tuberculosis, the use of essential oils brings about a lowering of fever, a reduction in coughing, regaining of appetite, weight and strength, a normalization of blood counts and the disappearance of the tubercle bacillus and scar cavities.

Rosemary aids the production and evacuation of bile; the essences of lavender, mint, sage and thyme are also choleretic.

Garlic, hyssop, juniper, lemon, nutmeg, and onion are prophylactic with regard to the formation of biliary or urinary calculi.

Lavender, marjoram, lemongrass, cypress and anise have antispasmodic properties. A few drops of essence of tarragon on the tongue will instantly stop hiccoughs; some drops of essence of cypress on the pillow will rapidly control a spasmodic cough; lavender calms an over excited nervous system.

Most essences are stimulants. The essences of pine (needles), borneol, geranium, basil, sage, savory and rosemary energize the cortex of the suprarenal (adrenal) gland; anise excites the anterior pituitary body, as does mint; onion, garlic and lemon are tonics. Onion, cinnamon, borneol, savory and ylang-ylang can help those whose sexual faculties are waning, whereas camphor has anaphrodisiac properties. Chamomile, garlic, onion and cinnamon are sudorifics.

Garlic, onion, anise, lemon, juniper and thyme act against fermentation, the major role played by an intestinal infection is the flare-up of the majority of diseases. The daily ingestion of aromatics gives proper balance and functioning of the intestines.

Numerous essences are vermifuge (an agent that destroys parasitic worms). Without listing them all, some to mention are garlic, chamomile, lemon, thyme, onion, wormseed, bergamot, caraway, cinnamon and gerniol.

Sage, cypress and lemongrass have hormonal properties, the essence of cypress being a homologue of the ovarian hormone. These have a balancing effect on the endocrine glands and operate by energizing and giving them new impetus rather than taking over the functions of deficient glands. This means that aromatic essences play a role of prime importance in the sphere of physiological excitation therapy. The properties of onion with regard to normalizing glandular imbalance and obesity are well known.

Among those essences which normalize and promote the menstrual cycle (emmenagogics) mention should be made of rue, valerian, artemisia, basil, cinnamon, cumin, lavender, melissa, mint, savin, clary and thyme.

The following can lower blood pressure: lavender, aspic (by peripheral action in lowering superficial blood pressure) and marjoram (by a central mechanism). The essences of hyssop, rosemary, sage and thyme on the other hand raise arterial pressure by liberating adrenalin as a result of direct action in the area of the cortex of the adrenal glands.

The anti-diabetic properties of eucalyptus, onion and geranium could well be put to profitable use since, as American research has shown the incidence of diabetes is rising; in fact their use ought to become quite common.

Other plants with similar properties include leaves of walnut, myrtle, mulberry, olive, agrimony, burdock, knotgrass, goatsrue and figwort.

From a different viewpoint, aromatic essences have been compared to vegetable hormones, we have already seen that the essence of cypress seems to be the homologue of the ovarian hormone and that essence of pine needles, and other essences, will stimulate the cortex of the adrenal glands.

# Essential Oils and Means of Administration

<u>For External Use</u>

Utilizing them externally, essences are used pure, or as a form for soapy or watery aqueous mixtures. The can also be in a solution with an alcohol content, or a liniment, or in the form of localized bathing. Sometimes, they can also be used as in the form of enemas, douches, inhalations or even as aerosols. Finally, they can also be administered through injections. Some different mixtures of aromatic essences (whole and natural) in their emulsion forms can also be widely used in an ordinary soaking bath. For adults, such mixture contains the essence of rosemary, cypress, sage, lavender, and thyme; for the mixture for children, it includes the essences of savory, thyme, rosemary and lavender, and for the sake of elderly people such mixture could contain wild thyme, geranium, juniper, and lavender. The effects would be tonic and/or calming, balancing or decongestive and can be experienced after a few baths.

Awareness of the components of these marvelous essences simplifies why many cases of obesity, arthritis, cellulitis, muscular weakness, circulatory problems, nervousness, and insomnia are relieved from the aromatic baths that are taken.

The diffusibility of the essences means that they will act as vectors, i.e. agents of penetration. For a long time they have been produced in the form of creams, balms and lotions so that their active properties might be absorbed easily throughout the body. The action of seaweed baths is necessarily reinforced and completed by the addition of certain essences, which, like vegetable hormones, are complementary in any case. Practice has confirmed this theory, and various mixtures of aromatic herbs are now used in association with seaweed to maximize the effects of seaweed baths.

## For Internal Use

Utilizing them internally, these essential oils are distinctly used in forms of capsules, drops or most often, in honeyed water. These essences are uniquely given alone or in combination with other oils. It depends on the case, but the dosage can vary between five and twenty drops of essence (pure) administered several times a day, usually before or during meals. Alternatively, between twenty and twenty-five drops taken four times a day in warm water (half a glass) and then sweetened with honey may be used. Because of their powerful effects, it's important to use these essences in solutions that are very diluted.

Care should be taken when essences are used which contain ketones, for in certain doses they may be epilepsy-inducing in patients so predisposed. The essences of rosemary, fennel, hyssop, wormwood and sage fall into this category, whereas anise, burdock, Melissa, mint and origanum are, according to Cadeac and Meunier, liable to be stupefacient (induce drowsiness) under certain conditions.

# Gathering and Preserving Aromatic Plants

Aromatic essences in therapeutic use are generally given in the form of drops or pills. We treat ourselves no less everyday by using aromatic herbs and plants in cooking; or we may equally look after our health by taking infusions of aromatic plants.

Most of the time, when you mention the word "herb," it means the part of the plant that grows above the ground. Sometimes this means the entire plant growing above ground, but most of the time it means only the top half of the plant.

The therapeutic effectiveness of the plants depends greatly on the way they are gathered and dried. It is vital that they preserve their active constituents to the fullest extent possible.

To ensure this, they should not be dried in direct sunlight, a condition like a loft, an oven, or in a drying cupboard works best. Hanging in small bunches or laid on airy racks usually work best. Allow the plants to dry naturally, then store in containers that are airtight and dry conditions.

In general, herbs should be gathered when they are in flower. Never gather your herbs on a wet day. Always wait until several days after a rain before collecting the herbs. Herbs should be gathered after the dew has dried from the plants, but before the sun gets too hot. This is when they hold the most of their essential aromatic oils.

The leaves can be gathered when the plant is flowering. Hang up the stalks (upside down) in small bundles to air dry until the leaves are completely dry. You can then crumble the leaves, keeping only those leaves that retain a green color, then store in a dark, tightly closed container. The stems have little medicinal value, so these need not be kept. Make sure the bunches of herbs hang loosely, so there is a chance for the air to circulate between the leaves. You do not want any mold to form on the leaves.

Some herbs need to be oven-dried to ensure that they are dried as quickly as possible. This can keep the leaves from turning black. Basil is one of the herbs that needs to be dried quickly, to prevent that from happening. Place a thin layer of the herb on a cookie sheet. Put in a very low heat oven, about 150 degrees. Prop open the oven door with a spoon to release the moisture from the plants (be careful not to touch the spoon with your hand since it will be very hot). Turn the herbs and watch them carefully. Remove when it crumbles easily. Cool and store in an airtight container immediately.

The seeds of herbs are gathered when they are not quite ripe, just before the seed pods are fully opened. Pick the whole head of the plant and place it in a paper bag, leaving these to dry in the bag. Shake the bag occasionally to work the seeds loose from the pods. It is then simple to pick out the flower heads, leaving the seeds at the bottom of the bag when the plant is completely dry. Be sure to leave plenty in nature for re-seeding to happen.

The flowers of the herbs are collected just as they are beginning to open. These should be placed on a screen to dry. Lay them on a screen in a single layer and turn frequently until they are completely dry. They should retain a natural color, so keep only those that do keep their color.

When drying fresh elder flowers, please take the precaution of hanging them away from people, pets and living areas. These release a volatile gaseous oil that may cause dizziness or headaches.

Most roots and bark are collected in the fall, with only a few exceptions. One exception is the wild ginger root. This should be gathered in the spring. As ginger is necessary for cooking and medicinal purposes, I thought I would make special mention of that. After getting a good patch of wild ginger to grow, you will be able to judge how much you can harvest without destroying your whole patch. Start with digging only small sections of the plant up.

We need to preserve the wild plants around us. Never, ever gather all of the wild herbs that you find. You need to be sure to leave plenty of plants alive to keep the species healthy and able to continue to grow. When gathering wild seed, it doesn't hurt to plant a few seeds that you have gathered. I try to leave the stronger and healthier plants where I find them. The stronger plants ensure that there will be more healthy plants in the future.

If you can't find any sources from which to buy bark, gather the bark yourself by pulling it off the tree by hand (only small amount). It is inner bark is the portion that is used, after the rough, outer bark is removed. The inner bark will tend to come off in strips.

Place the bark on a drying rack or screen, in a warm, well-ventilated room and allow to dry as quickly as possible. Low humidity is a must when drying the bark. Turn the bark daily to ensure even drying.

It must be stored in an airtight container to ensure that it does not develop mold or other harmful bacteria. Here's a way to help keep it free from bacteria and mold during storage: put several drops of camphor (a preservative) on an absorbent cloth. Place the cloth between two sheets of waxed paper and place it in the bottom of the container.

An attic is an ideal place to dry roots and bark, as it tends to stay warmer and dryer than the rest of the house. A greenhouse may also a good option as a place to dry roots and bark.

The roots are not too challenging to dry. After digging the roots, wash them thoroughly with a small scrub brush to remove all traces of soil. Drain well and slice the roots crosswise or lengthwise in thin pieces. Spread them on a screen in the attic or greenhouse, turning them occasionally to ensure thorough drying. Remember, roots and the bark need to be dried as quickly as possible to ensure a healthy product.

Always date and label the tins or jars in which you store your herbs. In this way, you can keep track of which herbs you have and how fresh they are. Roots can be kept for 3-4 years. The leaves and flowers can be stored successfully for several years, but will most likely need to be replenished yearly, due to frequent use of these. Fleshy roots, such as dandelion and burdock, should be replaced annually.

I frequently run out of the herbs that I use to make infusions because we drink them quite often, both for pleasure and for tonic purposes. I never know quite how much to preserve; that part is experimental to find our family's annual usage and most likely this will be true for you too. After a couple of seasons, you'll soon know what you use in large quantities and make it a point to preserve more of that. The bee balm and licorice mint, as well as the other mints, seem to get used up pretty fast around our place.

I keep my cooking herbs separate from my medicinal herbs. Some of them do overlap, but this is convenient, because I don't run out of any one herb as fast as I might otherwise. However, organize your herbs in a way that makes sense for you.

If, during the winter, I find I'm using large quantities of some of the herbs, I plan to plant larger beds of them in the spring, or if I don't grow them myself, I make a note to gather or purchase those. Planning your herb garden beds is a wonderful winter pastime. It also helps to make your greenhouse work a little less hectic, as you know exactly what you need to start planting in early spring, and can prepare as needed. I used to forget to plant several of the plants that I wanted to grow until I started making my lists ahead of time.

# Infusions or Decoctions

Plants are given in the same dose, whether fresh or dried; fresh plants are heavier and their properties more active.

- One pinch equals 2 to 3g
- One teaspoon equals 5g
- One tablespoon equals 10g
- One handful equals about 30 or 40g

Unless otherwise stated, the quantities are for adults. For children, prepare in the same way and then dilute as follows:

- At 1 year old: 1 part infusion to 4 parts water
- 1-3 years: 2 parts infusion to 3 parts water
- 3-5 years: 3 parts infusion to 2 parts water
- 5-10 years: 4 parts infusion to 1 parts water

When treating adults and of course, more especially children, individual susceptibilities (including possible allergic reactions) have to be taken into account.

When boiling water is required, the plants should be placed in cold water first, and then brought to a boil.

It is best to drink the infusions unsweetened; or if sweetened, then with honey or stevia rather than sugar.

If no specific time is given, the expression "give one boil" signifies boiling for a few seconds, then removing from heat and leaving to steep as directed. As a general rule, roots, stalks and bark should be boiled for 5 to 10 minutes. "One boil" is the correct method for whole plants, leaves, seeds and flowering tops. Flowers are infused (i.e. boiling water is poured on them).

You are to use enamel pans rather than pans made of bare metals. All other utensils used should be either made of glass or wood.

# Plant Preparation: Definition, Methods And Its Uses

**Alcoholic tincture**: Liquid obtained when a fresh plant is kept in alcohol for considerable time; more specifically, in a quantity of alcohol five times the weight of the plants.

**Aromatic baths**: put 500g aromatic compounds (q.v.) into a sachet (250g for children). Pour 1 - 2 gallons of boiling water and plant leaves to infuse for 10 to 15 minutes in covered vessel. Then add to the bath and fill tub to make water comfortable for the body. Soak and enjoy! Here is a guide to the indications of the different herbs you might want to try.

- juniper: recommended for arthritis and rheumatism

- lavender: sedative (for nervous complaints and insomnia). Indicated also for delicate or run-down children. Alternate with baths of pine, rosemary and seaweed.

- marjoram: tonic (similar to baths of thyme)

- pine: also fortifying. Recommended also for rheumatism and gout (foot baths may be used to treat excessive sweating of the feet)

- rosemary: fortifying, especially for children. Also beneficial in cases of rheumatism and weak eyesight

- sage: fortifying. Beneficial in cases of rheumatism

- thyme: again fortifying and in addition, indicated in

cases of arthritis, rheumatism, gout and chronic pulmonary conditions

- turpentine: anti-rheumatic

**Aromatized water**: aromatized distilled water (e.g. aromatized or distilled orange-flower water).

**Baths of combined essences and seaweed**: The practice of combining in the same bath both seaweeds of certain types of aromatic herbal compounds has, by giving the body the benefit of their different properties, extended the range of applications considerably, thus saving time. We may include here obesity, cellulitis, lymphatism, prolonged convalescence, anemia, chronic rheumatism, poor circulation, states of demineralization, premature aging, menopausal problems, problems associated with normal aging and certain skin conditions.

**Compounds**: The term given to essences or plants sharing the same properties (diuretic compounds, sudorific compounds, etc).

**Decoction**: Solution obtained by prolonged boiling of a plant (in a covered vessel). The plant is put in cold water, brought to a boil and boiled for 10 to 20 minutes. Bark and roots require longer boiling times than stems and leaves require.

**Embrocation**: Sprinkling a part of the body with an appropriate liquid which is then rubbed into the skin.

**Extract**: Substance obtained by partial evaporation of an aqueous, alcoholic or ethereal solution of a plant.

**Fomentation**: Application of a heated liquid, either by hand or with the aid of sponge, brush or flannel.

**Friction rub**: embrocation and friction rub meaning basically the same thing.

**Fumigation, Dry**: burn one or more plants over glowing embers.

**Fumigation, Moist**: the aromatic steam obtained by boiling one or more plants in water.

**Infusion**: The solution obtained by steeping a plant in boiling water for a few minutes (from 5 to 15 minutes, depending on the plant).

**Intract**: Special extract only obtainable from a plant which has preserved its original composition.

**Lotion**: Boil one or more plants in water and pass through fine muslin used in washes.

**Maceration**: Solution obtained by steeping a plant in cold water, wine, alcohol or oil to extract is soluble principles. This may take a few hours or several days, sometimes several weeks, depending on the case.

**Mustard compress**: Dip a piece of gauze in warm water, squeeze it out and spread on a flat surface. Sprinkle over it a layer of mustard powder. Apply to the affected part and leave it in place for about ten minutes from the moment the patient begins to feel it stinging slightly.

**Oils**: Half fill a wide-mouthed jar with dried plants or crushed roots and top off with olive or other vegetable oil. Allow to macerate for three weeks at a mild temperature, stirring from time to time. Decant into a flask. Obtained in this manner are the following medicinal or culinary oils:

- Chamomile oil: used in friction rubs for aches and pains

- Oil of St. John's wort: for pains and burns

- Oil of thyme, bay and rosemary: for grilling meat

**Ointment**: Preparation for external use, generally consists of a greasy base (oil, or fat) with or without active principles.

**Plant Juices:** Plants can also be ingested in the form of juice, especially good in a blender or vitamix with other fruits and vegetables. Listed below are some plants good for that use.

- *Juice of bitter and aperitive plants (biliary complaints):*
  - angelica (green stems) – 1 small handful
  - fumitory – 2 large handfuls
  - wild pansy – 2 large handfuls
  - chicory – 2 large handfuls
  - dandelion – 2 large handfuls
- *Juice of bitter and tonic plants (debility):*
  - peppermint – 1 small handful
  - speedwell – 2 large handfuls
  - lesser centaury – 2 large handfuls
  - marsh trefoil – 2 large handfuls
  - hops (green stems) – 2 large handfuls

- *Juice of anti-scorbutic plants (scurvy-mouth ulcers):*
    - scurvy grass – 3 large handfuls
    - shepherd's purse – 2 large handfuls
    - watercress – 2 large handfuls
- *Juice of refreshing plants (diuretic):*
    - purslane – 1 handful
    - sorrel – 1 handful
    - lettuce – 1 handful
    - white beet – 1 handful
    - viper's grass (black salsify) – 1 handful
    - dandelion – 1 handful

**Rob**: A sudorific and depurative syrup.

**Sinapism** (Mustard pluster): A mixture of mustard powder and water which is applied to the skin as a poultice to provoke a counter-irritation.

**Simple syrup**: A compound obtained by dissolving 3/4 cup sugar in 1/2 cup hot or cold water. Therapeutic ingredients are incorporated as required.

**Soft extract**: Evaporation is stopped at the point when the product has the consistency of honey.

**Spirit (of aromatic plants)**: Liquid obtained by distilling alcohol on a plant.

**Tincture:** Liquid obtained by dissolving the active constituents of medicinal plants in a suitable liquid (e.g. water, alcohol, ether).

From the point of view of antisepsis, to take one example, it is surprising to note the disfavor which has dogged aromatherapy through the decades which separate us from the initial work of Chamberland in 1887.

As research and experiment continue in the future concerning plants and their uses, more knowledge will be available to us. Even at present we nevertheless possess, in aromatherapy, a priceless tool.

This is all the more true since the effect of the essences is not limited to curing or alleviating. Aromatics have always played a healing part in the maintenance of health through the ages. By the changes they bring to the body, they can act as agents against a great variety of diseases, especially when used regularly and properly.

# Essential Oils and Some of Their Uses

Below you will find a list of different essential oils and some of the conditions they are helpful for.

*Aniseed*:

- aerophagy, flatulence
- nervous dyspepsia, nervous vomiting
- infantile colic
- migraine with nausea and vertigo
- palpitations, false angina pectoris
- asthma, bronchial spasm, cough, difficulty in breathing
- painful menstrual periods
- lacteal insufficiency

*Basil:*

- nervous debility (mental fatigue)
- anxiety, nervous insomnia
- gastric and intestinal spasm, painful digestion
- whooping cough, spasmodic cough
- migraine, some types of vertigo

- gout
- very light menstrual periods
- paralysis, epilepsy
- external use: loss of sense of smell due to chronic catarrh

*Bergamot*:

- general antiseptic and antispasmodic
- loss of appetite, dyspepsia
- intestinal colic
- intestinal parasites

*Borneo Camphor (borneol)*:

- prophylaxis and treatment of infectious diseases, influenza
- depressive states and debility (stimulates cortex of adrenal gland)
- convalescence

*Cajuput*:

- enteritis, dysentery
- cystitis, urethritis
- chronic pulmonary diseases (bronchitis, tuberculosis)
- laryngitis, pharyngitis

- gastric spasm
- asthma
- nervous vomiting
- hysteria, epilepsy
- painful menstrual periods
- rheumatism, gout
- intestinal parasites
- external uses: chronic laryngitis, rheumatic neuralgia, sores, skin diseases

*Chamomile:*

- loss of appetite
- migraine
- neuralgia (chiefly facial)
- painful teething in infants
- menopausal problems
- vertigo, insomnia
- painful digestion, stomach and intestinal cramps
- stomach ulcers, intestinal ulcers

- anemia
- nervous depression, convulsions
- scanty or painful menstrual periods
- influenza headaches
- intestinal parasites (roundworm, threadworm)
- intermittent fevers
- external uses: conjunctivitis, inflammation of the eyelids, inflamed skin conditions, eczema, herpes, boils, pruritis, sores, burns, rheumatic pains, gout

*Caraway:*

- nervous dyspepsia, gastric spasm, indigestion
- loss of appetite
- flatulence, aerophagy
- cardio-vascular erethism
- intestinal parasites
- difficult menstrual periods
- lacteal insufficiency
- external use: mange (in dogs)

*Cinnamon:*

- debility
- fainting
- sluggish digestion, gastric pain, flatulence
- digestive spasm, spasmodic colitis
- diarrhea, putrefactive fermentations
- uterine hemorrhage, haemoptysis (spitting blood)
- very light menstrual periods, leucorrhoea
- impotence, frigidity
- intestinal parasites
- external uses: scabies, lice, wasp stings, contusions

*Clove:*

- general physical and mental debility, amnesia
- impotence
- difficult digestion, dyspepsia, flatulence, diarrhea
- pulmonary diseases (tuberculosis)
- prevention of infectious diseases
- intestinal parasites

- preparation for childbirth
- malignant conditions
- external uses: toothache, sores, ulcers, scabies, lupus, insect repellent

*Coriander:*

- aerophagy, flatulence, painful digestion
- loss of appetite
- digestive spasm
- external use: rheumatic neuralgia

*Cypress:*

- hemorrhoids, varicose veins
- ovarian disorders (painful menstrual periods, uterine hemorrhage)
- menopausal problems
- whooping cough, spasmodic cough, aphonia (loss of voice)
- spasms
- influenza
- enuresis
- rheumatism

- irritability
- malignant conditions
- external uses: hemorrhoids, offensive sweating of the feet

*Eucalyptus:*

- diseases of the respiratory tract: acute and chronic bronchitis, cough,
- influenza, pulmonary tuberculosis, gangrene, asthma, pneumonia
- diseases of the urinary tract: various infections, colibacillosis, cystitis
- diabetes
- various feverish complaints and infections: measles, scarlet fever
- (prophylactic): cholera, malaria, typhus
- rheumatism, neuralgia
- intestinal parasites (roundworm, threadworm)
- migraine
- general debility
- external uses: sores, burns (cicatrising), lice, mosquito repellent, domestic disinfectant

*Fennel:*

- flatulence, sluggish digestion, gastralgia (stomach pains)
- aerophagy, loss of appetite, nervous vomiting
- oliguria, urinary stones, gout
- very light menstrual periods
- pulmonary diseases, influenza (prophylactic)
- lacteal insufficiency
- intestinal parasites
- external uses: congestion of the breasts, bruises, tumours, deafness

*Garlic:*

- prophylaxis and treatment of infectious diseases (epidemics of influenza, typhoid, diphtheria)
- asthma, emphysema (modifies bronchial secretions)
- diseases of the respiratory tract: bronchitis, tuberculosis, pulmonary gangrene, whooping cough, influenza, colds
- arterial hypertension
- arteriosclerosis, senescence (aging)
- rheumatism, gout, arthritis

- urinary stones
- gonorrhoea
- dysentery, diarrhoea, intestinal infections
- intestinal parasites (roundworm, threadworm, tapeworm)
- malignant conditions (preventive, by anti-putrid intestinal action)
- external uses: corns warts, verrucas, callouses, wounds, ulcers, scabies, tinea, deafness, earache, rheumatic, neuralgia, insect bites, cold abscesses

*Geranium:*

- debility (resulting from deficiency of cortex of adrenal gland)
- gastro-enteritis, diarrhea
- uterine and pulmonary hemorrhage (decoction of leaves)
- sterility
- jaundice
- diabetes (decoction of leaves)
- urinary stones
- gastric ulcer
- cancer of the uterus

- external uses: sores, burns, congestion of breasts, inflammation of mouth and tongue, sore throat, tonsillitis, facial neuralgia, opthalmia, impotence, lumbar and gastric pains, scurf, dry eczema, lice

*Ginger:*

- loss of appetite
- painful digestion, flatulence
- diarrhea
- scurvy
- external use: rheumatic pains

Hyssop:

- asthma, hay fever, pulmonary emphysema, difficulty in breathing
- chronic bronchitis, cough, influenza
- loss of appetite, painful digestion
- gastralgia, colic
- rheumatism
- leucorrhea, light menstrual periods
- urinary stones
- intestinal parasites

- malignant conditions
- external uses: dermatosis, eczema, sores, bruises

*Juniper:*

- general debility; organic lassitude (sluggish digestion)
- prophylactic of contagious diseases
- diseases of the urinary tract: albuminuria, oliguria, gonorrhoea, cystitis
- gout
- rheumatism, arthritis
- urinary stones
- diabetes
- dropsy, cirrhosis
- arteriosclerosis
- leucorrhea, painful and difficult menstrual periods
- flatulence
- external uses: after-effects of paralysis, sores, ulcers, weeping eczema, acne, toothache (Cade oil), domestic disinfectant, canine mange

*Lavender:*

- irritability, spasm, insomnia

- diseases of the respiratory tract: asthma, bronchitis (acute), spasmodic, cough (whooping cough), influenza, etc.

- eruptive fevers, infectious diseases

- scrofulosis (ganglions)

- general physical and mental debility, anxiety, melancholy

- infantile debility

- migraine, vertigo, hysteria, epilepsy, after-effects of paralysis

- enteritis (diarrhea), dyspepsia, sluggish, digestion, gastric atony

- cystitis

- oliguria

- leucorrhea, light menstrual periods

- intestinal parasites

- external uses: the treatment of wounds of all descriptions, burns, acne, eczema, lice, scabies, insect bites, animal and snake bites, used also in inhalations and as a domestic disinfectant

*Lemon:*

- various infections, infectious diseases, epidemics (prophylaxis and treatment)
- debility, loss of appetite
- rheumatism, arthritis, gout
- gastric hyperacidity, stomach ulcers
- arteriosclerosis, hypertension
- varicose veins, phlebitis, capillary fragility
- plethora, hyperviscosity of the blood
- ascites (dropsy of the abdomen)
- urinary stones, gallstones
- demineralisation, growing pains, convalescence, pulmonary tuberculosis, tuberculosis of the spine (Pott's disease)
- anemia
- scurvy
- jaundice, hepatic congestion, hepatic deficiency
- painful digestion, vomiting
- hemorrhage (nasal, gastric, intestinal, renal)
- diarrhea

- malaria, feverish conditions
- intestinal parasites
- equally: asthma, bronchitis, influenza, haemophilia, gonorrhoea, syphilis, headache
- external uses: inflammations of mouth and tongue, thrush, buccal syphilides, infected and putrid wounds, verrucas, warts, herpes, tinea, scabies, eruptions of various kinds, boils, insect bites

*Lemongrass:*

- difficult digestion
- enteritis, colitis
- upsetting of sympathetic nervous system and resulting disorders (spasm, palpitations, vertigo, etc.)
- insufficiency of milk production
- external use: lice

*Marjoram:*

- (properties similar to those of peppermint and thyme)
- general debility
- digestive spasm (aerophagy), flatulence
- respiratory spasm

- nervous debility, mental instability
- migraine
- anxiety, insomnia, tics
- external uses: rheumatic neuralgia, head colds

*Niaouli:*

- chronic and fetid bronchitis, pulmonary tuberculosis
- whooping cough
- rhinitis, sinusitis, otitis
- tuberculosis of the bones
- intestinal infections (enteritis, dysentery)
- urinary infections (cystitis)
- puerperal infections (after childbirth)
- external uses: sores, atonic wounds, burns, fistulas, pulmonary diseases, laryngitis, whooping cough, coryza (head cold)

*Nutmeg:*

- chronic diarrhea
- difficult digestion
- halitosis, flatulence

- debility
- gallstones
- external uses: rheumatic pains, toothache

*Onion:*

- general debility, physical and mental fatigue
- growing pains
- retention of liquid in the system
- oliguria
- rheumatism, arthritis
- excess urea in blood
- obesity
- gallstones
- diabetes
- difficult and sluggish digestion
- diarrhea, intestinal fermentation
- genitor-urinary infections
- respiratory diseases (colds, bronchitis, asthma, laryngitis)
- glandular imbalance

- arteriosclerosis, senescence (retards)
- prostatitis, impotence
- lymphatism, rickets
- scurvy
- intestinal parasites

*Orange Blossom:*

- cardiac spasm, palpitations
- chronic diarrhea
- insomnia

*Origanum (Oregano):*

- loss of appetite
- sluggish digestion, gastric atony
- aerophagy (digestive spasm), flatulence
- chronic bronchitis, irritating cough
- pulmonary tuberculosis
- asthma
- acute or chronic rheumatism, muscular rheumatism
- amenorrhea (absence of menstruation)

- external uses: rheumatic pains, lice

*Peppermint:*

- general debility
- indigestion, gastric atony, aerophagy
- stomachache, acidity of the stomach
- flatulence, diarrhea, cholera, gastro-intestinal poisoning
- gastric spasm and colic
- liver complaints
- nervous vomiting
- palpitations, vertigo
- migraine, tremors, paralysis
- difficult and painful periods
- asthma, chronic bronchitis
- impotence (mild action)
- intestinal parasites
- external uses: headache, migraine, toothache, scabies, mosquito repellent; used in inhalations

*Pine:*

- all diseases of respiratory tract (asthma, bronchitis, tuberculosis, tracheitis, etc.)
- urinary diseases (pyelitis, cystitis, prostatitis)
- infections in general
- gallstones
- impotence
- rickets
- stomachache, intestinal pains
- external uses: pulmonary complaints; generally in baths (rheumatism, gout, etc.)

*Rosemary:*

- general debility, physical and mental fatigue, amnesia
- chlorosis, lymphatism
- asthma, chronic bronchitis, whooping cough
- intestinal infections, colitis, diarrhea
- flatulence, difficult digestion, stomachache
- rheumatism, gout
- hepatic disorders, jaundice, gallstones, cirrhosis,

- cholecystitis
- excess of cholesterol in the blood
- painful periods, leucorrhea
- migraine
- disorders of the nervous system
- cardiac complaints of nervous origin
- vertigo, fainting, hysteria
- external uses: sores, burns, lice, scabies, tonic, and aphrodisiac baths; rheumatism

*Sage*:

- (a general tonic to the system)
- debility, (convalescence, etc.), nervous debility
- dyspepsia, sluggish digestion, loss of appetite
- diarrhea
- nervous complaints: trembling, vertigo, paralysis
- chronic, bronchitis, asthma
- nocturnal sweating in tubercular patients and convalescents
- profuse sweating of hands and armpits
- oliguria

- lymphatism
- hypotension
- painful and light periods, menopause
- preparation for childbirth
- sterility
- intermittent fevers
- lactation (to dry up)
- external uses: leucorrhea, thrush, stomatitis, throat infections, toothache,
- atonic wounds, eczema, insect bites and stings (wasps, etc.), tonic baths

*Sandalwood:*

- specific for urinary infections: gonorrhoea, cystitis, colibacillosis
- chronic bronchitis
- persistent diarrhea
- impotence

*Savory:*

- painful digestion
- mental fatigue
- impotence
- gastric pains of nervous origin
- flatulence, intestinal fermentations
- intestinal spasm
- diarrhea of all kinds
- intestinal parasites
- asthma, bronchitis
- eye strain

*Tarragon:*

- upsets of the sympathetic nervous system (aerophagy, hiccough)
- loss of appetite, sluggish digestion
- stomach-ache, nervous dyspepsia
- flatulence, putrefactive fermentations
- rheumatic neuralgia
- painful and difficult periods

- intestinal parasites

*Terebinth:*

- chronic and fetid bronchitis, pulmonary tuberculosis
- urinary infections, cystitis, urethitis
- leucorrhea
- hemorrhage (intestinal, pulmonary, uterine, nasal)
- gallstones
- spasms (colitis, whooping cough)
- rheumatism, gout, neuralgia, sciatica
- migraine
- intestinal parasites (especially tapeworm)
- chronic constipation
- epilepsy

*Thuja:*

- cystitis, enlarged prostate, pelvic congestion
- rheumatism
- external uses: verrucas, warts, condylomas, adenoids (as a gargle)

*Thyme:*

- general physical and mental debility, nervous debility, anaemia

- chlorosis

- asthma

- spasmodic cough (whooping cough, etc.)

- pulmonary diseases

- sluggish digestion

- intestinal infections

- diseases resulting from chill (influenza, colds, stiffness, shivering, sore throat)

- infectious diseases

- intestinal parasites (hookworm, roundworm, threadworm, tapeworm)

- aids the circulation; indicated for unnatural suppression of periods

- leucorrhoea

- also aids sleep

- external uses: dermatoses, boils, wounds, lice, scabies, vaginal douches, sprays (generally in association with other essences), care of teeth and gums, rheumatism

*Ylang-ylang:*

- hypertension (high blood pressure)
- tachycardia (acceleration of heartbeat)
- intestinal infections
- purulent secretions
- impotence, frigidity

# Make Your Own Essential Oils

We'll be looking at several methods for making your own essential oils from raw plants, although there may be other ways as well.

Some people opt to make their essential oils by using a steam distiller. They can be a homemade version, or for a fairly reasonable price one can be purchased. One example, so you can see what one looks like, is found on Amazon at

http://www.amazon.com/2000ml-Steam-Distillation-Essential-Extractor/dp/B002065JL2

If you use a purchased distiller, you'll follow the manufacturer's guidelines for its use.

Although it is outside the scope of this book to teach how to build your own distiller, the basic components needed in any unit would be the following:

- Heat source

- Holding tank which holds the water and the plants on some type of false bottom or grate, similar to a vegetable steamer

- Condenser - collects steam and cools it

- Separator - this portion separates the essential oil from the water vapor

You'll first want to decide what kind of essential oil you want to make, and then gather your plants. Most of the herb's essential oils are found in the plants' veins, hairs and oil glands. You can distil either fresh plants or dried. Be sure the plants are free from ıdes and other chemicals because you don't want to distil those ... your oil. By drying a plant first, while it does reduce the amount of oil in the plant, it can also increase your final yield per batch, due to the fact that you can fit a lot more dried plant material into the distiller than you can fresh plants. It is best to distil as soon as possible after drying for optimum conditions.

It takes quite a large quantity of plant material to make essential oil. Put your water in your still, then put your raw plant material on a rack or false bottom just above the water in the holding tank. The plants can be stacked quite high on the grate or false bottom, as long as it does not block the steam outlet area.

Be sure to use enough water to complete the distillation process (this varies according to the plants you are using), although in worst case scenarios, you could add more boiling water if needed. Don't let the holding tank dry out. Bring the water to a boil, and continue until the plant has yielded up its oil, which most do at around 100 degrees Celsius or 212 degrees Fahrenheit, the herb will turn brown. This process could take anywhere from half an hour up to 6 hours, depending on the plant and quantity you are processing.

A process known as hydrodistillation is very similar at this stage. The difference is that the plant material is actually in the water, and not in a false bottom or rack above the water. This is used for processing powdered roots, bark or delicate flowers.

Keep a watch on the process, after a bit the water vapors and oil will begin to enter the condenser area, and then into the separator. Make sure you don't run out of water in your holding tank at this point, and you'll want to add more ice to the cool water in the condenser portion so that it keeps cooling the distillate. Other than this, this part is fairly hands off.

Once the distillation process is finished and the oil is cool, you may want to filter the oil through a clean cheesecloth before pouring into your jar, although this step is optional. You do want to put your oil into a clean, dark colored glass jar as soon as possible, then store in a dark, cool place.

At this point, some people add a bit of alcohol like vodka or gin to the essential oil to help aid as a preservative and also help dilute the essential oils a bit, as they are very concentrated.

Others opt to dilute them in the glass jars with a carrier oil of some type. Popular choices are sweet almond oil, grapeseed oil and olive oil, but that is up to the individual. One thing to consider however is that carrier oils may have a shorter shelf life than the pure essential oils do.

Hydrosol is the water that was used for the distillation process that collected in the separator. Some are useful as a separate product on their own, such as lavender or rose water. If you don't plan to use this hydrosol, you can either throw it out, or pour it into the holding tank for your next distillation batch.

Now, to show you another method of making your own essential oils, without a distiller. Sometimes this process is known as enfleurage.

Gather your equipment and materials needed.

- 1/2 cup olive oil, sweet almond oil or grapeseed oil
- 4 cups plant material (raw or fresh), tightly packed
- Wide mouth glass mason jar & lid

- Wood mallet or something similar to crush plants

- Wooden spoon

- Large ziploc bag

- Cheesecloth

Place your plant materials into the ziploc bag, removing as much air as possible before sealing. Using the mallet or a rolling pin, bruise and crush the plants somewhat; not into a powder or anything, just to break them up some.

Put the plant material into the clean mason jar. Pour your oil over the herbs, and stir well with the end of a small wooden spoon, ensuring the plants are completely contacting the oil. Put the lid on and set in a warm location for 2 days. Every few hours give it a good shake.

When the 2 days are up, filter through a cheesecloth and return the oil to the jar. Add another batch (4 cups tightly packed), of the same plant materials used the first time around and repeat the process, allowing this to 'cure' another 2 days.

Repeat this process 2 more times only these times use 2 cups of plant material instead of 4, for a grand total of 4 times.

When the 4th cycle has completed, strain and pour into dark colored glass jars, date and label. These will keep for about a year, store in a cool dark area.

# Preparing Your Medicine Chest

Now that you have grown, harvested, and dried your herbs - and have a basic knowledge of their many uses - you should prepare your own herbal medicine chest. You do not need a large supply of herbs. Your medicine chest may be designed to hold only a few remedies, but it is important that you have a special place for them, and that they are kept out of the reach of children and pets.

As you become more familiar using different herbal medicines, you will get some idea of which herbs you will need to keep on hand. It's a personal decision; no one can tell you what you need. If someone in the family has a tendency to get chest colds, you would prepare some of those remedies, or at least have on hand different herbs needed to create those remedies so you can treat them at the first sign of illness. Sometimes, by treating a particular illness early, we can limit the severity or duration of it.

I know what tonics, salves, and tinctures I need for my family. By keeping some of these available, I can be prepared for just about any illness or accident. Here is a list of some of the remedies that I keep on hand. I find that I use some frequently and others hardly at all.

All of the recipes for these remedies are found later in the book.

1. The menthol camphorated oil is the first thing I use on a strained muscle, soreness or arthritis. It's also my first choice for easing chest tightness.

2. In keeping a good assortment of the tinctures on hand, we use the valerian tincture the most. Use it to treat different skin rashes, headaches and nervousness. If a feeling of a

cold is coming on, try the antibiotic tincture and the rosemary tincture. Use the calendula to clean cuts and scrapes, but almost any of the tinctures are good for that, so don't worry too much if you run out of calendula tincture.

3. Always have several of the salves on hand. Use the Balm of Gilead salve to treat burns and scratches.

4. Keep an earache tincture ready for use. Use it when you have ear problems and to keep you comfortable.

5. Always keep a cough syrup on hand, and in autumn try to keep a supply of cough drops made. They are delicious. We suck on those even when we don't have a cough.

6. Keep several kinds of herbal capsules prepared for home use. Take the menopause capsules if someone is going through that stage, along with the capsules for poor circulation. To save time, and to have them ready when you need them. Try to make at least a two-month supply of the capsules at one time.

7. In the cabinet, place all the vitamin supplements that you might need to take during bouts of illness. Also stock some herbs to make remedies for other, less common needs.

8. The dried herbs found in tea or infusion remedies are effective and easy to use, so just keeping them on hand is enough to enable you to treat many personal illnesses. It may take a little time to get the supplies you need, but it is well worth the effort.

Keep all the cooking herbs in the kitchen spice cabinet. The other herbal preparations designed for bath or personal care should be kept in the linen closet or bathroom. The personal care products are used daily and, of course, should be kept where they will be used.

It doesn't take as much time as you might think to make herbs and herbal products for daily use. Even if they did take a lot of time, making them for our health's sake would be worth it. There is a lot of self-satisfaction in using nature's bounty.

# Which Part of the Herb is Used?

*Acacia (Acacia senegal)*

The exudation (serum fluid) is the part used. Removes phlegm from the throat and bronchia. Used for conditions for the respiratory and digestive organs.

*Alkanet (Alkanna tinctoria)*

The root is the part used. Used for blood disorders, liver and gallbladder problems.

*Allspice (Linedera benzoin)*

Fruit, leaves and twigs are used. Breaks fevers.

*Angelica (A. atropurpurea)*

Roots, seeds and leaves are used. Expectorant for colds and coughs. Also treats kidney disorders and aids the digestive system. Caution: be careful not to mistake poison hemlock for Angelica because even though they are nearly identical, every part of hemlock is deadly even in very small amounts.

*Anise (Pimpinella anisum)*

The leaves and seeds are used. Anise is good for colds and flu. Licorice or anise hyssop is a great to relieve fever. It is used as a digestive aid. It can be added to recipes for teas that include unpleasant tasting herbs. Anise adds a nice licorice flavor to any tea.

*Apple (Pyrus mallus)*

The whole fruit is used. Dried apple tea is an excellent diuretic. Aids in elimination of toxins from the system.

*Asparagus (Asparagus officinalis)*

The shoots and the roots are used. Warm tea made from asparagus is used as an excellent diuretic. Drink every 2-3 hours.

*Balm of Gilead (Populus candicans)*

Of this tree, it is the closed buds that are used as an expectorant for both bronchial problems and chest troubles.

*Basil (Ocimum basilicum)*

Basil is used as a mild sedative, help with digestion and headache relief. It is the leaves that are used. Some people can be sensitive to it however.

*Bee Balm (Monarda didyma)*

All plant parts can be used.. Bee balm is used as an antiseptic, because it contains thymol. It's also used to stimulate spleen and liver.

*Blackberry (Rubus spp.)*

The fruit, roots and leaves and used for various sicknesses. Dissolves deposits in both the kidneys and the alimentary system.

*Black Alder (Prinos verticillatus)*

Both the fruit and bark are useful for gallbladder and liver issues.

Cleanses the body of mucoid toxins.

*Boneset (Eupatorium perfoliatum)*

The upper portions of this herb are most commonly used and are cleansing on all organs of the body. It's both a muscle relaxant and helps eliminate mucus from bronchial, liver, bower and alimentary systems.

*Borage (Borago officinalis)*

Both the flowers and leaves are used. It has a cooling type taste and is nice in teas. Often used to help with depression symptoms. If the flowers are made and used as a tea, a common use is for colds and fevers.

*Calendula (Calendula officinalis)*

Calendula flowers are an ingredient used for many different ailments. It's useful for treating wounds as it contains antibiotic qualities. It can also be used for flu, stomach issues, cramps, and to help reduce a fever.

*Catnip (Nepeta cataria)*

The flowers and leaves can be helpful in treating flatulence and colic.

*Celery (Apium graveolens)*

If a tea is derived from celery (only use fresh celery), it help ease stomach discomfort.

*Chamomile (Matricaria chamomila)*

The upper parts of the plant, and flowers are used for its sedative and calming effects. It also is useful for cramps, gastrointestinal problems and headaches.

*Chicory (Cichorium intybus)*

Chicory flowers are used as a diuretic, general tonic, and a sedative.

*Clary Sage (Salvia sclarea)*

Seeds and the leaves of the plant are used for eye troubles, kidneys and liver. It's also good for stomach ailments like colic and nausea.

*Cleavers (Galium aparine)*

This herb is an effective diuretic, with the whole plant being used.

*Coltsfoot (Tussilago farfara)*

Leaves are what are used in this herb, which helps to detoxify and eliminate those toxins from the body.

*Comfrey (Symphytum officinale)*

This works well as an expectorant, emollient and demulcent, with the leaves and roots being used. Caution should be exercised however as this plant has some controversy surrounding it, regarding it being a possible carcinogen.

*Corn silk (Zea Mays)*

This is effective in cleansing the urinary system, a diuretic and tonic for the whole body. Good for fighting bladder or kidney infections.

*Dandelion (Taraxacum officinale)*

Works well for gallbladder and liver issues and a general tonic. The leaves and roots are most commonly used.

*Elder (Sambucus canadensis)*

A tea made of the flowers works well as a diuretic, and on the common cold. The fruit, leaves and flowers are used.

*Eyebright (Euphrasia officinalis)*

This can be made into a rinse for eye health, and the seeds can be used to help combat kidney stones.

*Fennel (Foeniculum vulgae)*

Fennel is good to help promote healthy digestion, and increase breast milk production. All parts of the plant can be used.

*Fenugreek (Trigonella foenum-graecum)*

The seeds of this plant help calm the intestines and lining of the stomach.

*Ginseng (Panax quinquefolia)*

The root of ginseng has been a very popular remedy for centuries. If used as a general tonic, it helps overall health and is said to be an aphrodisiac.

*Goldenseal (Hydrastis canadensis)*

This aids both liver and stomach problems and the root is what is used.

*Horehound (Marrubium vulgare)*

The leaves and flowering tops are used for stomach and bronchial troubles. It also helps with colds and sore throats and works as an expectorant.

*Hollyhock (Althea rosea)*

Not only is this plant beautiful, the leaves and roots are useful. The leaves, if cooked can be used as a side dish, or left raw in salads. Good to use when battling a cold, or if one is vulnerable to kidney stones.

*Irish Moss (Chondrus crispus, and gigartina mamillosa)*

This plant must be dried for use and is helpful for kidney and bronchial problems. Sometimes it is used in cough syrups.

*Kelp (Fucus vesiculosis)*

Kelp is helpful for goiters and to purify the blood.

*Kidney Beans (Phaseolus vulgaris)*

By using the pods and beans to make a tea, it makes a diuretic. This also aids the kidneys.

*Lavender (Lavandula angustifolia)*

Lavender has made uses, but mainly the flowers are used. It's known for its calming and sedative qualities. Helpful also for headaches and relieving tension.

*Lemon Balm (Melissa officinalis)*

If a tea is made with the leaves, not only does it have a sedative effect, but helps to reduce fevers and regulate menstruation in women.

*Lemon Verbena (Aloysia triphylla)*

Prepare a tea of the leaves to calm an upset stomach. It also is good for the intestines, and good when battling the flu or colds. It has a sedative quality and helps reduce fever.

*Licorice (Glycyrrhiza glabra)*

The root of the plant is what is used, most commonly to aid women during menopause, since it possesses estrogen type of characteristics. It can also be used for bronchial and blood problems.

*Marsh Mallow (Althaea officinalis)*

It is the root of the plant that is used, and it helps ease inflammation and irritations of the alimentary and urinary systems. It also will help calm a ticking or hoarseness of the throat and aid with bronchial problems.

*Mullein (Verbascum thapsus)*

While all of the plant can be used, the leaves and flowers are the most commonly used parts. Helps with fighting colds due to its antibiotic qualities, and good for bronchial troubles as well.

*Nettle (Urtica dioica)*

Both the upper parts and leaves of the plant are used to help relieve pain due to arthritis. Sometimes also used for weight loss.

*Nutmeg (Myristica fragrans)*

In tiny doses, nutmeg can help digestion and stomach problems.

*Pansy (Viola tricolor)*

The entire plant can be used as a tonic for the heart, asthma and colds. It can also be eaten in salads, while adding beauty to the dish.

*Parsley (Petroselinum crispum)*

The whole plant is used and is a wonderful diuretic. If a tea is made, it's been used to help kidney issues.

*Pennyroyal (Hedeoma pulegiodes)*

It is the leaves that are used and helps calm upset stomachs and is a mild stimulant. Because of that it's sometimes used to help fight menstrual cramps.

*Peppermint (Mentha piperita)*

The flowering tops and leaves are what is used. Peppermint dispels hardened mucus from the bronchial and alimentary systems. It's also used for stomach problems and colds.

*Plantain (Plantago major)*

It's the leaves and roots that are used on this plant, which carries antiseptic qualities and help remove toxins from the body.

*Pokeweed (Phytolacca americana)*

The roots, berries and young shoots are used in this plant, and extra caution needs to be used with this plant. It's a very powerful purge. It mimics the effects of cortisone, an adrenal hormone, which stimulates the endocrine system. Keep away from children!

*Pricky Lettuce (Lactuca virosa, and l. scariola)*

The gum and leaves are used, as it is a strong sedative and used to help insomnia.

*Purslane (Portulaca oleracea)*

Everything part of the plant above ground can be used, as a diuretic that helps cleanse the kidneys.

*Raspberry (Rubus idaeus)*

The fruit, roots and leaves are used. If a tea is made using the leaves, it stimulates the kidneys, and helps uterine muscles relax. The roots have an astringent property, and also some antibiotic value as well.

*Red Clover (Trifolium pratense)*

It is the flowering tops that are used, both as a tonic and blood purifier. Many skin problems can be resolved when drinking a tea of made of this regularly.

*Rose Hips (Rosa canina)*

The flowers, leaves and hips are used as a wonderful tonic for the blood. Rose hips contain Vitamin P which helps to resolve ruptures of small blood vessels, it also contains lots of Vitamin C.

*Rosemary (Rosmarinus officinalis)*

Rosemary is a popular herb used in cooking and can be used as an astringent. It helps muscles to relax, is used to treat depression and headaches.

*Sage (Salvia officinalis)*

It is the leaves that are used to help remove toxins from the body, and stimulates the kidneys. It has a sedative effect and can be useful for headaches. It is used to treat colds and helps remove catarrh in the bronchial and alimentary systems. Do not take in excess! Do not use if breastfeeding.

*Sassafras (Sassafras albidum)*

It is the bark of the root that is used to purify blood and thin it. It's also useful for the kidneys.

*Sheep Sorrel (Rumex acetosella)*

The parts of the plant above ground are what is used for blood disorders, cleanses the urinary system and reduces fevers.

*Shepherd's Purse (Capsella bursa-pastoris)*

The whole plant can be utilized. It stimulates uterine muscles. It can also be used to treat diarrhea due to the astringent qualities. It helps stop bleeding so useful when that is needed.

*Skullcap (Scutellaria laterifolia)*

The plant parts growing above ground is used, mainly for its sedative qualities to treat insomnia, headaches and nervous disorders.

*Slippery Elm (Ulmus fulvus)*

The inner portions of the bark are what are used. As an expectorant, it calms the bronchial and alimentary systems.

*Solomon's Seal (Polygonatum officinale)*

This herb is used as a diuretic that has strong expectorant action to aid with bronchial problems. It is the root portion that is used.

*Spearmint (Mentha spicata)*

It is the flowering tops and leaves that are commonly used for treating colic, as a diuretic and problems with the alimentary system. Not to mention and fabulous tasting tea!

*Sweet Woodruff (Galium odoratum)*

This is such a beautiful smelling herb! It's the top part of the plant that is used as a blood purifier and tonic for liver and the heart. It also aids with upset tummies.

*Tag Alder (Alnus serruluta)*

Both the bark and the cones are used, most commonly as a diuretic.

*Thyme (Thymus vulgaris)*

In this popular herb the whole top portion of the plant is used. It helps for bronchial issues, and has antiseptic qualities as well as being a stimulant for cleansing urinary and alimentary systems. Not to mention very useful in cooking.

*Valerian (Valeriana officinalis)*

It's the root of valerian that is used. It has a powerful calming effect and used to treat insomnia and nervous disorders.

*Vervain (Verbena hastata)*

The whole plant is used and possesses both expectorant and diaphoretic qualities, useful for chest issues like colds with fevers.

*Violet (Viola odorata)*

Violets are one of the richest sources of vitamin A out there. The roots, leaves and flowers are used, both as a mild sedative and a general tonic. The root is good for stopping diarrhea and to calm stomach pain.

*Watercress (Nasturtium officinale)*

Loaded with vitamin C, the whole plant is used. Its rich in mineral content like iron, manganese, copper, sulfur and calcium, which makes is very good or anemic problems and a good overall tonic.

*Wild Ginger (Asarum canadense)*

This herb is both a diuretic and stimulant, with the root portion being used. It is useful for the kidneys and as a general tonic for the body.

*Wild Strawberry (Fragaria virginiana)*

*and Garden Strawberry (Fragaria vesca)*

The berries, leaves and roots of the plants are used. If a tea is made with the leaves, it is dense in minerals like potassium, iron, sulfur, sodium and calcium so very healthy overall. It is sometimes used to treat gout, and for the urinary and alimentary systems.

## *Willow (Salix spp.)*

The bark, twigs and leaves are used and contain salicylates and salicin, which was used for the first aspirin medications. Good pain relieving qualities for general pain and also during bouts of flu or colds.

## *Woad (Genista tinctoria)*

The roots provide us with natural blue dye and the leaves are good for the liver and gallbladder. The whole plant can be used.

## *Wild Yam (Dioscorea villosa)*

It is the root of the plant that is used; it has an estrogen quality so is popular for women in menopause. It may also be used for asthma and other bronchial problems.

## *Yarrow (Achillea millefolium)*

Good for treating feverish conditions, the whole herb can be used. It also contains salicylates and silicin so has pain relieving properties. The roots help aid blood disorders. It is mineral rich with calcium, iron, sodium, sulphur and potassium for great overall health. Due to its astringent qualities it can also be used externally for sores and wounds.

# Preparations of Essential Oil Capsules, Salves, Syrups and Tinctures

In this section, you can learn how to prepare your own capsules, salves, syrups, and tinctures. I've also included many different recipes that use different ways of preparing the herbs.

Preparing salves and liniments for future use is a good idea. If you prepare them in advance, you will have them on hand for emergencies or for everyday use. Of course, there will always be recipes that might not be prepared ahead of time, but their ingredients can be placed in tightly closed containers and clearly labeled. Always use sterile containers and be sure to clearly label each with the contents, use, dosage and date. Small dark glass jars work well, or plastic P.E.T. cosmetic jars also, make sure they are BPA free.

It may take time to build up a nice supply of the kind of herbs needed for your remedies, but it is well worth the effort. If you are going to have a big supply of herbs, you must have containers in which to store them. I collect antique tin canisters and keep dried herbs in them.

It is important to put a preservative in the recipes that you plan to store for indefinite periods of time. If honey is used in the recipe, that will be sufficient, as honey is a great preservative. If you are not using honey, adding the oil from several vitamin E capsules to your herbal mixtures is another way to help preserve them. Gum benzoin (which is a balsamic resin that can be purchased) is called for in some of the recipes. This is a preservative and you will not need to add any other preservatives if you are using it.

*Preparing Capsules*

Herbs or essential oils can be ingested in capsule form, tinctures, or teas. Many times capsules are chosen for their ease to take while we are away from home, such as work. They are sometimes used because some herbs and tinctures are extremely bad tasting.

Empty gelatin capsules can be bought at a local pharmacy or health food store. Usually there are many sizes offered, but the size #00 is used most frequently. To fill them, pull them apart, then put your herbs in the largest portion, and put the top on to close it. Root herbs can either be bought in powdered form, or dried and blended to a fine texture with a food processor, then if necessary ground to a finer powder with a pestle and mortar. It must be a dry and very fine powder. The leafy parts of the plants can be put in a food processor to be powdered.

If you were using an infusion (tea remedy), and the dosage is 3 cups a day, then you would need 1 capsule 3 times daily.

If you are already on a medication, or need to take a medication to control your blood pressure, please do not substitute these capsules for your regularly prescribed medication; consult your physician or a naturopath doctor.

*Blood Pressure Capsules*

In a food processor mix 1 Tablespoon each of the following herbs in dried form: spearmint, elder flowers, stinging nettle, yarrow, chamomile, and powdered valerian. Place into capsules. These were chosen for the following reasons:

Stinging nettles helps to not only flush water and toxins from the body, but also aids in weight loss. It also is useful for arthritis, and to stimulate hair growth.

Spearmint is an effective diuretic and helps with inflammation trouble of the kidneys or bladder.

Elder is sometimes also known as boretree. It is helpful for removing mucus in the bronchial tubes; thereby good for treating chest congestion, coughs and colds. It is also a diuretic and detox agent for the body.

Valerian is useful for its known calming affects, yet it is also a stimulant and diuretic for the kidneys.

Chamomile is used due to its calming properties, a good way to help lower blood pressure to keep as calm as one can.

Yarrow was chosen because it's a good source of potassium, as diuretics tend to flush potassium out of the body, this helps to counteract that effect.

*Menopause Capsules*

Because menopausal symptoms are the result of the depletion of estrogen hormones, you need to make a recipe that will nourish both the adrenal glands and the ovaries. The adrenal glands carry on the production of this hormone when the ovaries are missing.

For women dealing with menopause and its symptoms try making a blend of herbs having estrogens qualities. Popular choices are licorice root, wild yam root and black cohosh root. The goal is not necessarily to replace the missing estrogen, but trying to get the body to make its own substitute version.

For this recipe you'll mainly be using the roots of the herbs, please use in a powdered form so they can be easily made into capsules. For skullcap and chamomile you'll be using the plant tops. Combine 1 Tablespoon of chamomile, motherwort, valerian, wild yam root, black cohosh, skullcap, and licorice root and blend well in a food processor. You will then place this mixture in capsules. Ingest 2 of these three times a day until symptoms back off, then continue with 2 capsules per day.

Below you'll see why each of these herbs were chosen for this recipe.

> Valerian due to is calming effects on the whole body.

> Black cohosh relaxes muscles, calming to nerves and general tension, and provides estrogen type qualities.

> Chamomile was chosen for the sedative traits, and will help ease gastrointestinal issues and cramping.

> Motherwort is a wonderful general tonic overall, supports the nerve system, relieves headaches and eases menstrual pain.

> Wild yam possesses a molecule called diosgenin, which is an estrogen similar type. It is reacted to by the body as an estrogen, making it very useful during menopause and pre-menopause.

> Licorice root supports the adrenal glands and also contains estrogen type qualities.

> Skullcap is useful to helping sleep problems, headaches and anxiety.

*Flu Capsules*

This recipe is good to help knock the punch out of the flu or colds. In a food processor blend 1 Tablespoon of each herb: elder flowers, yarrow, verbena, powdered valerian root, peppermint, verbena, horehound and boneset. Put this mixture in capsules, taking 2 every 3 or 4 hours until symptoms are greatly reduced.

> Yarrow is chosen because it contains salicylic acid derivatives that offer pain relief and help to reduce fever. It also fights infections and inflammation.
>
> Elder flowers help to promote sweating, which also helps fevers to reduce.
>
> Boneset is a good tonic for the whole body, a diaphoretic, and muscle relaxant and helps to cleanse the body.
>
> Verbena helps to fight nausea and calms the intestines and stomach as well as helps bring down fevers.
>
> Peppermint also helps to ease nausea and aids digestion.
>
> Valerian will help a person relax and get the extra rest needed to recuperate. It also helps to stimulate the kidneys to help flush the toxins out of the body.
>
> Horehound helps to cleanse mucus from the bronchial system.

*Lung Congestion and Sinus Treatment Capsules*

The use of herbs is an important component to help promote faster healing in the body. They help provide vital nutrients, detoxify and at times helps to reduce symptoms of specific ailments or diseases.

Herbs that have a stimulating effect helps to increase production of various hormones and enzymes, help the kidneys in removing toxins and wastes from the body. Some herbal plants kill bacteria, or other destructive organisms.

When dealing with congestion, the body in order to cope and protect sensitive mucous membranes, produces phlegm and mucus. This recipe will help break up congestion. Use 2 capsules every two hours for three days, then after that, 2 capsules a day until congestion is gone.

In a food processor, add 1 Tablespoon each of thyme, slippery elm, comfrey and fenugreek. Insert into capsules.

This is why these herbs are chosen in this recipe:

> Fenugreek helps to reduce inflammation and is a germicidal agent for the lungs.
>
> Slippery elm helps the mucus and phlegm to move easier out of the respiratory system by causing it to ball up. It also provides soothing and healing qualities for the lungs.
>
> Thyme has great antiseptic traits as well as expectorant actions.
>
> Comfrey root has been commonly used for congestion issues for many years by reducing inflammation and breaking up congestion in the lungs and chest area.

*Memory Retention Capsules*

Poor circulation can be caused by high cholesterol and other factors like environmental toxins and poor diet. Many times there may also be problems with poor memory, varicose veins, and hemorrhoids.

Try this recipe with a good vitamin B complex source.

In a food processor add 1 Tablespoon of each: lecithin, apple pectin, cayenne pepper and butcher's broom. Mix well and insert into capsules. Ingest two each morning and evening. After a month, take 2 capsules daily.

> Butcher's broom for centuries has been used to treat circulation troubles and prevention of blood clots following a surgical procedure.

> Lecithin breaks down fat deposits within the circulatory systems, allowing it to be flushed from the body.

> Apple pectin attracts heavy metals and pollutants in the blood so they can be flushed out. It also aids in lowering cholesterol levels and regulating the bowels.

> Cayenne pepper attacks bacteria and carries vital nutrients in the body to where they are needed faster to promote healing. Not only can it help dissolve cholesterol deposits, it can help lower blood pressure as well.

*Preparing Salves*

Salves need a preservative because they are often used for cuts and wounds and as such need to be free from bacteria. A good preservative to use is tincture of benzoin, which you can purchase from your local drugstore. It is inexpensive and necessary for the preparation of your salves. Choose stainless steel, glass, or earthenware when you are looking for bowls or containers; they should be airtight and sterile.

It is helpful to know what the basic ingredients of a salve are. The ingredients used to make the salves are: the herbs you plan to use, an oil, beeswax, and the preservative. The best kind of oil to use is olive or sesame. Do not use the drying oils, such as soybean and linseed.

*Basic Salve Recipe*

Salves are very useful to have on hand in your medicine chest and make excellent gifts as well. They can be put in small jars, and they will keep for years. When making your salve, consider the use you'll be applying it for, then choose the appropriate herb or herbs for that need.

To make a basic salve recipe in general, you'll heat the oil in a glass pan or stainless steel, just below the boiling point. You can make this in an oven if you prefer that over stovetop. Add your herbs and simmer about 3 hours. If you use fresh herbs, keep the lid off for the first half hour so the water can evaporate from the plants. If you are using roots or bark, put these ingredients in the oil first and simmer for 1 1/2 hours before adding the other herbs. Keep the cooking temperature low and keep it covered while cooking.

When the time cooking is done, strain; and then add beeswax to the amount of 1 1/2 ounces for each 2 cups of oil used. Stir well, then add 1/2 teaspoon tincture of benzoin as a preservative, for each 2 cups of oil used, then mix. Test for texture by putting a small amount of the liquid salve in a spoon and put in the refrigerator. If it's too thin, add a bit more beeswax and test again until you get it to the right consistency. Pour into your jars, then label.

*General Salve Recipe*

Combine 2 Tablespoons each comfrey, calendula and plantain leaves, to the above basic method. This salve works well for both pain relief and healing properties of skin conditions and wounds.

*Pain Relief Salve Recipe*

Mix 2 Tablespoons of each herb: wormwood, chickweed and yarrow to the above basic method. This is a great pain relieving salve and promotes healing of skin while fighting infection.

*Preparing Syrups*

As you become more experienced in working with herbs, you will find the confidence to create your own recipes. To help you do that, below are recipes that include explanations of why each herb is included. Categories are also listed such as stimulants, diuretics, expectorants, astringents, nervines, and tonics. Herbs from one category can be substituted for another form from the same category. Of course, not all of the herbs in each of the categories are equal to each all of the herbs in each of these categories are equal to each other as far as their potency and their secondary effects, so a little research will help you select the appropriate herbs from the categories.

When making cough syrups, the herbs should be dried, and these mixtures generally are boiled then strained. Honey is then added and it's allowed to simmer for roughly an hour. Flavoring (cherry oil is a popular choice) is added when the concoction has cooled.

Here are popular types of herbs that are used for cough syrups;

Aromatics: these are known for their amazing scents. Some are sassafras bark, mint, marjoram and fennel.

Demulcents: these provide the action of softening or soothing, usually helping various mucous membrane areas. Popular choices are hollyhock, Iris moss, slippery elm, balm of Gilead, honey, mullein and mallow.

Stimulants or activators: this action increases a function temporarily, such as a diuretic increasing urine production, or a diaphoretic increasing sweating.

*Basic Cough Syrup Recipe*

Combine the following dried herbs: 1 teaspoon each of elecampane, boneset, slippery elm, wild cherry bark, yarrow, and coltsfoot. Add 1/2 teaspoon of thyme, 2 teaspoons of Irish moss. Add 1 Tablespoon each of peppermint, mullein and balm of Gilead.

Mix this dried mixture with 4 cups of water and boil until only 2 cups of liquid remain. Strain and return liquid to pan. Add 2 cups of honey and simmer for 30 minutes. Cool and bottle. Dosage is 1 teaspoon every hour while needed.

*Preparing Tinctures*

What exactly is a tincture? It is a highly concentrated liquid extracted from an herb and may be taken internally, or used externally in general. It is important to know the specific qualities of the herb you will be using; however, some are meant only for external use, while others are intended to be taken orally. Make sure that you only ingest herbs that you know for sure are safe to be used in that way.

## How to Make Your Own Tincture

For a basic tincture recipe, combine half a cup of the herb you want to make a tincture of, with 2 cups alcohol into a large glass jar; that may be gin, rum, vodka, or even glycerin or some other type of vegetable oil. The medicinal alkaloids and oils from the herbs will be extracted by the alcohol. Shake this mixture once per day, allowing it to age for 2 weeks. Strain and pour your newly made tincture into dark glass containers, clearly labeled. An average dosage would be 10 - 25 drops for adults, and 5- 10 drops for children.

## Antibiotic Tincture

For this recipe, combine 2 cups of nasturtium flowers and leaves, 2 cups garlic cloves, 2 cups rosemary stems and needles with 4 cups of vodka. Shake daily and allow to age 2 weeks, then strain. This is good for fighting infection and dosage is 1 full dropper every two hours for a few days.

## Clove Oil Tincture for Toothaches

Clove oil has for many years been very popular in relieving pain from toothaches. Combine equal parts olive oil and whole cloves, then allow it to steep for 4 weeks. Strain and bottle. Apply with a Q-tip to the area of the toothache, and see a dentist.

Cinnamon oil can be made the same way as well. To infuse a lovely scent into your home, you can use a few drops of these oils into a pan of simmering water.

*Earache Tincture*

Use a small glass jar and fill with mullein flowers. Pour olive oil over the material until just covered. Allow to steep in the sun for 1 week. You will want to shake this mixture once daily. Strain and it's ready for use; drop 3-4 drops in the ear as needed to soothe pain, then cover with a moist, warm wash cloth.

*Wound Care Tincture*

Combine 2 Tablespoons of the following ingredients; yarrow, nasturtium flowers & leaves, and crushed garlic. Add to this 1/2 Tablespoon of Echinacea root and 2 cups vodka. Shake this mixture daily and allow to steep for 2 weeks. Strain, then bottle in a dark bottle.

This is wonderful to use to externally to clean scrapes and cuts to help prevent infections. You can also ingest it orally with 1/2 dropper full every few hours for three days. This is good for fighting colds and infections.

The nasturtium helps to remove mucus from the body and works as an antiseptic, the garlic works as a natural antibiotic, yarrow has an antiseptic quality as well as pain relieving properties. Echinacea root helps cleanse the lymphatic system, works as an antibiotic and a blood purifier.

*Calendula Tincture*

Combine 2 cups of olive oil with 1 cup of calendula flower petals and allow to steep for 2 weeks, shaking daily. Strain and add a couple drops of tincture of benzoin (which acts as a preservative) and store in a sterile bottle.

This mixture is very handy to have on hand at all times, it can be used on chapped skin and lips, to treat sores and clean wounds. Calendula also has styptic qualities in that it helps stop bleeding.

*Valerian Root Tincture*

This tincture has many uses including as a sleep aid, treating poison oak or ivy, on cold sores and other skin problems. It is also useful for sinus or tension headaches, and sore muscles.

To make mix 1/2 cup valerian root and 2 cups vodka, allowing it to steep 2 weeks. Strain and put into a sterile bottle. Dosage for adults is 1/2 dropper full once every 4 hours. This can also be put into a #00 capsule to ingest if desired.

# Essential Oils For Beauty Treatments

Beauty products are important to our physical and mental health. Many commercial beauty products contain artificial chemicals and these chemical substances do penetrate the skin. Every time we apply these commercial products to our body, we are absorbing substances through our skin that we would never dream of putting in our mouth.

The natural recipes are simple to make. Try different ones to find the types that are effective for you. Keep in mind that if your skin has a tendency to be dry, you would not want to use too many astringents. Keep in mind any allergies you might have as well. Before making any remedy, try each of the herbs to be used on a small patch of skin as a test before using. You might not be aware of some of the allergies that you perhaps have (or have recently developed).

Remember, there is beauty and majesty in natural simplicity.

*Basic Cleansing Cream*

Add 2 Tablespoons beeswax, 2 Tablespoons herbal infused water (see below), 3/8 cup olive oil, 4 Tablespoons lanolin and a couple drops of essential oil for scent if desired. In a double boiler, melt beeswax and lanolin on low; once this has melted add olive oil. Remove heat and add scent if using, and the herbal infused water. Stir constantly until it has cooled, it will thicken as it does. Put in a screw top jar.

*Herbal Infused Water*

Mix 3-4 Tablespoons of your favorite herb (suggestions below) with 1 1/4 cup boiling water in a glass bowl. Allow to steep for 30 minutes, then strain, bottle and chill. This is useable for a week. You'll want to use this chilled as a toner for skin.

- Comfrey: smooth wrinkles
- Chamomile: tones up muscles
- Thyme: astringent, to help clear acne

  Rosemary: tightens skin
- Fennel: clears up brown spots
- Lemon Balm: smooth wrinkles
- Mints: excellent astringents for oily skin

Directions: Use the cleansing cream to clean your face twice daily. Massage a small amount on your face, then place a hot clean cloth on the face, then gently wipe the cleanser off. Rinse with cool water, then apply the herb infused water with a cotton ball onto skin as a toner.

*Essential Oils On Hair Care*

Hair styles come and go. The hair has to be healthy to withstand the stress we put it through daily. Diet plays an important part in keeping our crowning glory healthy. Simplify your diet and your hair benefits. Use some of these recipes as a start of getting a healthier hair.

*Hair Shampoo*

Put 2 tablespoons of white oak bark into 1 cup of water. Bring to a boil and reduce heat to simmer. Simmer for 20 minutes. Strain and add to 2 tablespoons of liquid castile soap. Now add 3 tablespoons of the herb soap to 1 teaspoon of honey and 1 beaten egg. Shampoo hair. Rinse well with apple cider vinegar rinse. This one is great for older people to use.

*Hair Rinse*

Pour 4 cups of boiling water over 2 tablespoon of the chosen herb. Cover and let stand 30 minutes. Strain and use as a hair rinse. It is a simple matter to make a hair rinse from any of the following:

- Sage: a good conditioner
- Fennel: also conditions
- Parsley: clears up dandruff
- Chamomile: Lightens hair, promotes growth
- Rosemary: Darkens hair, leaves a delicious fragrance
- Nettle Leaves (use dried): excellent to treat dandruff

*Herbal Shampoos*

Put 2 tablespoons dried soapwort, 1 tablespoon chamomile flowers, and 2 teaspoons borax in a large jar or container made out of pottery or chinaware. Pour 2 ½ cups of boiling water over the herb mixture and cover tightly. Let steep for several days. Shake the container every once in a while. Strain and discard the herbs. This will not be as soapy as a commercial shampoo, but its cleansing qualities are undeniable. Add a few sprigs of lavender or lime blossoms before covering to give a natural, delicate fragrance. Soapwort is nothing more than wild sweet William, so it is easy to grab a few handfuls to make the shampoo.

*Oily Hair Rinse*

Use this as a final rinse for oily hair. Put ½ cup of rosemary into 1 ½ cups of water. Bring to a full boil, then simmer for 15 minutes. Let sit 24 hours, covered. Strain, bottle, and use daily for one week. Thereafter, use at least once weekly.

*Shampoo Substitute*

Beat an egg and massage into scalp twice each week. Rinse with vinegar water, then rinse with plain water. This is a good treatment for your hair. Leaves hair shiny and healthy.

*Wild Chamomile*

Make an herbal infusion by pouring 4 cups boiling water over 5 tablespoons chamomile flowers. Cover and steep 30 minutes. Strain and add ½ cup castile soap flakes. Makes 4 cups of shampoo. This is the favorite shampoo around many households. You can purchase the castile soap flakes from any of the companies that sell herbs. It's easy to make and easy on the hair.

*Yucca-root Shampoo (also called soapweed)*

Dig or purchase the yucca roots. Chop into small pieces and pulverize into a pulp (using a hammer or blender). When the substance has changed from white to pale amber, it is ready to use. You can dry for later use by spreading the material on a clean surface in the sun until all moisture has evaporated. The pulp should no longer feel sticky.

When using this shampoo, make sure that your hands are free from grease, or the shampoo won't lather. Place a small amount of the root in a cheesecloth bag. Wet and lather to wash hair. Leaves the hair shiny and silky.

If you must use commercial shampoo, then follow this recipe: use a ratio of 2 tablespoons of apple cider vinegar to 2 cups of water to make a final rinse for hair after shampoo. This counteracts the alkaline effect of commercial shampoo.

*Essential Oils For Skin Care*

Taking care of our skin is very important. The skin, in fact, is our first defense against any invasion of foreign matter that can be harmful to our system. The skin is considered a third kidney because we excrete toxins through the just as we do through the kidneys. We also ingest many chemicals and toxins through the skin, so it is important that we pay attention to what we use to clean, soothe, and heal it. The skin also plays an important part in regulating our body temperature.

Most injuries to our skin are easy to treat, yet essential. The first step for any puncture or wound is cleansing it immediately, and seeking medical assistance if necessary. Keeping the area clean during healing prevents many problems from developing later on.

Some skin problems are indicative of internal problems, such as an improper diet. Diet plays an important part in caring for our skin. If we stick to a simple, natural diet and use only natural products to clean or protect us, we will have a much healthier immune system; one that is better able to deal with the viruses or bacteria that we come into contact with daily. Keeping the immune system healthy should be the major goal in seeking a healthy lifestyle.

One of the first ways you can begin to live a healthy lifestyle is to make your own soap. Many people would like to live healthier, but believe that it is difficult to do. The whole procedure takes about 1 ½ hours from start to finish. I make it as I need to, and only have to do so a couple of times per year.

In this homemade soap there are no artificial chemicals and the ingredients are simple. Your basic tools will be; a half gallon jar, a couple flat containers that can be lined with plastic wrap, an iron or enamel pot, a thermometer (needs to register low temps 95 - 98 degrees), wide mouth glass jar and a wooden spoon.

Here are some important guidelines when making the soap:

1. Prepare the containers either by lining them with plastic wrap or greasing them with olive oil. Do this before making your soap.

2. Always use stainless steel, iron or enamel pots or pans, never aluminum.

3. When curing the soap don't allow it to be in a drafty area as this will negatively affect the finished soap. Cover it with thick newspaper, then a folded blanket on top of that for several days for beautiful looking soap.

4. Ensure your containers that you'll be using as molds are a minimum of 1 1/2 to 2 inches thick.

5. If you choose to add scent to your recipe, add it right before pouring into the molds. Any essential scented oil will work, usually about 2 Tablespoons for each batch, and adjust from there to your preference.

6. When making the lye solution in the wide mouth glass jar, do so carefully and with no children around. If possible, do this step outdoors; splatters can damage countertops, and outdoors gives optimum ventilation. Wear rubber gloves and do not breathe the fumes. Pour the lye very slowly, into very cold water. This will heat up while you are pouring the lye into the water. Stir carefully and slowly; you want to avoid all splatters. Continue stirring until lye is completely dissolved. Once this is ready, place the jar in a cold water bath in the sink (or a larger pan) to reduce the temperature down to 90 - 95 degrees. When that temp has been reached, you can slowly pour the lye solution to oil.

If you do splatter lye on the skin, rinse immediately with water, and rinse with vinegar.

*Basic Soap Recipe*

For the lye mixture, add 5 cups cold water to your wide mouth glass jar, then slowly add 1 1/2 cups of lye until completely dissolved.

In an iron, stainless steel or enamel pan, slowly melt 6 pounds of lard. When the lard has melted, put the pan in a cold water bath to reduce the temperature to 120 - 130 degrees. You might want to have this close before starting the lye solution so you don't need to wait long on this.

When both the lard and lye are at correct temperatures, slowly pour the lye into the lard stirring carefully with a wood spoon, then keep stirring continuously for 30 minutes. Add the scent if you are going to, then pour carefully into the greased molds. Allow this mixture to cool overnight. The next morning, you'll need to cut the soap into individual bars and then begin the curing process, allowing it to rest for 2 - 3 weeks.

There are countless variations of soap recipes that can be made using different ingredients, such as different types of oils, butters, milks, textures and other items. Some people find making soap is a joy to accomplish, and turn it into an amazing hobby or business.

# Essential Oils For Tonics and Teas

In some cases, illness may be caused by a poor diet. We all need tonics to keep the body supplied with certain minerals and vitamins in order to keep our immune system strong and healthy. If the immune system is in good order, then it is able to fight off certain illnesses. Then, if we do pick up a bug, our bodies can respond to the invading organisms much faster and we are able to start the healing process more quickly. We may not be able to avoid an illness totally, but we may be able influence the length and severity of it.

Sometimes we are vulnerable genetically to specific diseases or conditions. When we are aware of those health frailties we can become more proactive to strengthen those areas to protect our health. Certain herbs can help us strengthen the body so it can do its job of repairing and healing faster in a healthy manner.

Natural remedies with herbs are not necessarily a quick cure. Often, the process is slower than we would like for a specific plant to work because many times its not only helping the body fight the known illness, but other possibly underlying conditions. Tonics also take time to work so we need to continue to give them the period of time needed to do the work.

In can be helpful to think of the use of herbs as preventative care for our bodies. The closer we can get to an optimum state of health, the better it can ward off disease, and other conditions of poor health.

Just as the herbs can help us be balanced internally, we must look at ways we can be balanced externally, in our daily lives. All the money in the world cannot take the place of your health, and this is where balance in your lifestyle comes into play. I'm sure you have heard it said that all work and no play makes Jack a dull boy. Well, all play and no work can do the same thing. There is no time in your life for everything: work, play, quiet time, pleasure, people, love, and many other joys. Be not a slave to any one activity and you will have some measure of control (and balance) over your life. Learn to stop and smell the roses. Even though that is old advice, it is still good advice.

No one else is as interested in preserving our health and the health of our families as we are. We know how we want our foods, and what we want in our foods better than anyone. When we preserve or prepare our own foods, we can take precautions to ensure that the foods and herbs are handled properly and in a hygienic manner. We can make sure that what we ingest is as natural as possible.

What could be more natural than adding tonics to our daily life? Tonics are beneficial to ingest year around. They can become part of your health-protecting diet. They can also be a great alternative energy boost to caffeine.

## *Tonics*

### *Adrenal and Respiratory Tonic*

Combine 2 Tablespoons of each herb; hyssop, marshmallow root, horehound and licorice root. Add in to this 4 cups of water and simmer until liquid is reduced by 1/4th, or reduced to about 3 cups. Strain. Drink 1/2 cup of this tonic every few hours, 1 day a week for a month. This mixture supports the respiratory system and provides nourishment for the adrenal glands.

## Adrenal Glands Stimulate Tonic

Place 1 Tablespoon of the chopped leaves and flowers of borage into 2 cups of boiling water. Allow to steep 10 minutes and then strain. You can add honey is desired. Drink several cups per day for 1 week. This is a good energy drink.

## Mental Concentration Tonic

Combine 2 Tablespoons of goldenseal, 8 Tablespoons rosemary, 5 Tablespoons yerba mate, 3 Tablespoons skullcap, 2 Tablespoons sage, and 1 Tablespoon cayenne pepper. Put 1 teaspoon of this mix into 1 cup boiling water, then steep 10 minutes. Strain and sweeten if desired. Drink this tonic twice daily for 2 weeks, and then reduce it to only once daily.

## Wild Strawberry Leaf Tonic

This general tonic is great for overall health and wellbeing. Dry wild strawberry leaves for use when not in season. Put 1 teaspoon of wild strawberry leaves into 1 cup of boiling water. Allow to steep 15 minutes, then strain and sweeten if desired. Drink 3 cups daily for 1 week.

## Violet Leaves Tonic

Here's another wonderful general tonic to use. Boil 8 cups of water, then add the peels of 2 oranges and 3 lemons, simmer for 15 minutes. Remove from heat then add 6 Tablespoons of violet leaves and flowers, and 6 Tablespoons of hops then steep an additional 15 minutes. Strain and sweeten if desired. Drink several cups daily or as often as desired. This one is good for the whole family.

*Indigestion Mix Tonic*

Combine 1 Tablespoon of each type of seed: coriander, caraway and aniseed. Crush 1 teaspoon of this mixture then pour into 1 cup boiling water. Allow to steep until cool, then strain and sweeten if desired.

*Blood Purifier Tonic with Sorrel*

Gather a large handful of sheep sorrel leaves and pour 2 cups of boiling water in a bowl. Allow to steep 15 minutes, then strain. Drink 2 cups daily for a week. This helps to cleanse the urinary system, aids inflammation, reduces fevers and helps skin problems.

*Blood Strengthening Spring Tonic*

Boil 4 cups of water, then add 2 Tablespoons of each herb; dandelion root, boneset, burdock root, and sarsaparilla, then boil for 15 minutes. Strain. Drink one glass 3 times daily for 3 days. This can be refrigerated and consumed chilled as well.

*Cardiac Tonic*

Combine 2 Tablespoons of motherwort, 2 Tablespoon calendula, 1 Tablespoon goldenseal, 4 Tablespoon cayenne pepper and 4 Tablespoons of hawthorn berries and mix together. Place 1 teaspoon of this mixture into 1 cup boiling water. Steep covered for 10 minutes, strain and sweeten if desired. Drink 3 times a day for 1 week.

*Menopause Tonic*

Add 1 Tablespoon of each of the following herbs; chamomile, gentian, hops, skullcap and motherwort. Place 1 teaspoon of this mixture into 1 cup boiling water and allow to steep 15 minutes. Strain, then sweeten if desired. Drink several cups each day for symptoms when needed. This is a very calming blend.

*Comfrey Energizing Tonic*

In a blender, add one can frozen orange juice and appropriate amount of water per the directions on the can. Add 2 comfrey tender, new leaves and blend well. Not only is this drink refreshing, it has an energizing effect.

*Costmary Tonic*

Take a handful of chopped costmary (sometimes known as bible leaf) leaves and add to 2 cups of boiling water, allow to steep 15 minutes. Strain. Drink 3 cups daily for a week. This is excellent for the liver.

*Dandelion Tonic*

Put 2 Tablespoons of dandelion flowers into 2 cups of boiling water then steep or 10 minutes. Strain and sweeten if desired. Consume 3 glasses a day for a week. This is a good, overall tonic which provides energy, vitamins and minerals.

*Feverfew Tonic*

Add 2 Tablespoons of dried feverfew flowers to 2 cups of boiling water then allow to steep 15 minutes. Strain and sweeten, if desired. Drink 1/2 cup twice for one day. This helps to stimulate the nervous system.

*General Tonic*

Steep 3 pumpkin blossoms in 1 cup boiling water for 10 minutes, then strain and sweeten. This gives many rich minerals and vitamins for overall health and wellbeing.

*Heart and Brain Tonic*

Place 3 Tablespoons of either dried or fresh wild rose petals into 2 cups of boiling water, steep 15 minutes. Strain and sweeten if desired. Drink 2 cups daily for a week.

*Heart Strengthening Tonic*

Take 1 Tablespoon of chopped ginseng, 1 Tablespoon of cinnamon into 2 cups of honey. Simmer for 30 minutes, strain and cool. Ingest by the spoonful a couple of times daily. This tonic helps increase blood circulation.

*Rose Hips Tonic for the Heart*

In 1 cup of boiling water, add 2 teaspoons of crushed rose tips, let simmer for 3 minutes. Strain and sweeten. Drink three times daily as often as needed.

*Heart Strengthening Violet Tonic*

Crush 2 teaspoons of violet leaves and add 1 cup of boiling water, steep 10 minutes. Strain and sweeten as desired. This can be consumed as often as you want.

*Hawthorn Berry Heart Tonic*

Put 3 Tablespoons of hawthorn berries into 2 cups of boiling water and allow to steep covered, overnight. While straining the next day, be sure to squeeze all the liquid from the berries. Drink a cup twice daily for a week.

*Honeysuckle Heart Tonic*

Boil 7 cups of water and add 1 cup grated honeysuckle root, reduce heat and simmer for 30 minutes. Strain then chill. Consume 2 cups per daily for a week.

*Nasturtium Flowers Internal Cleanser Tonic*

Add a handful of nasturtium leaves and flowers to 2 cups of boiling water and allow to steep 30 minutes. Strain and sweeten if desired. Drink 2 cups a day for 1 week. This tonic is helpful to both the digestive system and blood.

*Spleen & Liver Tonic Strengthener*

In 4 cups of water, simmer 1 1/2 cups honeysuckle leaves and 1/2 cup honeysuckle blossoms for 10 minutes. Strain, and drink twice daily, before meals for 1 week. This also helps when battling a cold to dry up mucus.

*Dandelion Root Live Tonic*

Boil 6 cups of water, 2 Tablespoons dandelion root chopped up, 2 Tablespoons senna leaves, 2 Tablespoons cinnamon bark, 2 Tablespoons chopped ginger root and 2 Tablespoons caraway seeds. Boil until liquid is reduced to 3 cups. Add 1 1/2 cups agave syrup or sugar and continue boiling for 2 minutes. Cool and strain, then store in refrigerator. Take 1 teaspoon several times a day for 1 week.

*Liver Tonic & Purifier*

In 2 cups of boiling water, add a small handful of fresh watercress, cover and steep 15 minutes. Strain and sweeten if desired. Drink 3 times a day for a week. This is a tonic for the alimentary and urinary systems.

*Sassafras Spring Tonic*

Boil 2 cups of water, add 3 teaspoons of sassafras bark or root, then allow to steep 15 minutes. Strain & sweeten if desired. Drink 3 cups daily for 1 week. This was commonly used in the spring for many years to add nutrients and minerals back into the body.

**Teas**

*Cinnamon Tea*

With cinnamon being a good stimulant that does causes a person to sweat, it's a good choice to drink when one has a cold. In 2 cups of water, add 6 cinnamon sticks and simmer 30 minutes. Strain and add honey or milk to taste. A very cozy beverage too!

*Hyssop Tea*

Hyssop tea is great to drink while fighting a cold and in particular congestion. Add 2 or 3 Tablespoons of hyssop leaves to a teapot full of water. Adding grated lemon and orange peel is a nice, nutritious touch as well. Steep 15 minutes, strain and sweeten. This tea also helps to reduce a fever.

*Peppermint Tea*

Combine 1 Tablespoon peppermint leaver, 1 Tablespoon elder flowers, 1 Tablespoon of feverfew and 1 Tablespoon of white yarrow. Pour 2 cups of boiling water over this herb mix and steep for 15 minutes. Strain and sweeten if desired. This helps as a pain reliever, dispels mucus and reduces fever and great when a person is battling a cold.

*Rice Tea*

Boil 6 cups of water, add 1/2 cup rice and simmer for 15 minutes. Strain then add a bit of honey and vanilla, and drink warm. This is great for helping nausea, vomiting, and to stop diarrhea quickly, making it very useful for bouts of the flu. It also tastes great and kids will love it too.

*Rosehip Tea*

This tea is a great vitamin C boost anytime. Pour 1 cup boiling water over 1 teaspoon of dried lemon peel and 1 teaspoon crushed rosehips, allowing this to steep 15 minutes. Strain and sweeten with honey.

*Sweating Tea*

Combine 1 Tablespoon each of the following herbs; boneset, thyme, mint, sage, verbena, catnip and white yarrow. You can substitute any of these if you want with elder flowers, linden, horehound or pennyroyal. In 1 cup of boiling water, steep 1 large teaspoon of the herb mix for 10 minutes. Strain and sweeten if desired. Drink a cup every 3 or 4 hours.

# Conclusion

Herbal plants can add so much value to our health and wellbeing, and yet we have only scratched the surface. With so many forms to make use of, and the combinations that can be created, it could well take a lifetime to study all there is to know and most likely even that wouldn't be enough time. It is my hope that this has provided some insight and whet your appetite to learn even more about how to incorporate herbs into your life.

If you enjoyed this book or received value from it in any way, would you be kind enough to leave a review for this book on Amazon? I would be so grateful. Thank you!

**Disclaimer**

All material in this book is provided for informational use only. Do not interpret it as medical instruction or advice. No action or inaction should be used based solely on the information contained in this book. Readers should get appropriate advice from their health professionals on any matter relating to their health. Additionally, some individuals can have allergic reactions to a specific herb that is not considered toxic.

Made in the USA
San Bernardino, CA
14 July 2016